EVALUATING
HEALTH
PROMOTION

A HEALTH
WORKERS
GUIDE

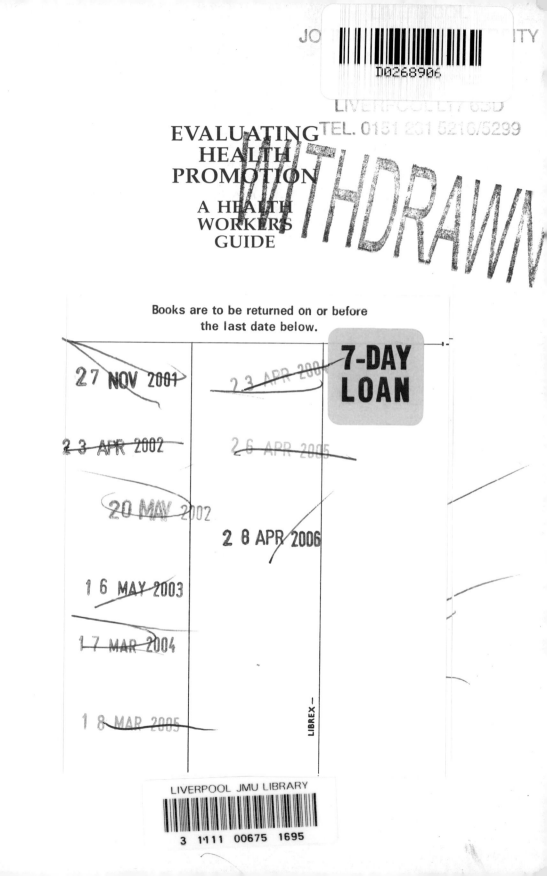

Books are to be returned on or before
the last date below.

**7-DAY
LOAN**

27 NOV 2001

2 3 APR 2004

2 3 APR 2002

2 6 APR 2005

20 MAY 2002

2 8 APR 2006

1 6 MAY 2003

1 7 MAR 2004

1 8 MAR 2005

LIBREX —

ALL ROYALTIES FROM THE SALE OF
THIS BOOK ARE DONATED TO THE
PUBLIC HEALTH ASSOCIATION OF AUSTRALIA
TO SUPPORT AN EARLY CAREER AWARD IN
HEALTH PROMOTION EVALUATION

EVALUATING HEALTH PROMOTION

A HEALTH WORKER'S GUIDE

Penelope Hawe
B.Sc. Psychology Hons, M.P.H.

Senior Lecturer in Health Promotion
Department of Public Health, University of Sydney

Deirdre Degeling
R.N., B.A., M.Sc

Director, Area Health Promotion Centre
Western Sydney Area Health Services

Jane Hall
B.A., Ph.D.

Director, NSW Centre for Health Economics Research and Evaluation
Department of Community Medicine, Westmead Hospital

with the assistance of
Alison Brierley
B.A.Hons

Department of Community Medicine,
Westmead Hospital

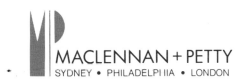
MACLENNAN + PETTY
SYDNEY • PHILADELPHIA • LONDON

First published 1990
Reprinted 1991, 1992, 1993, 1994, 1995

MacLennan & Petty Pty Limited

ACN 003 458 973

80 Reserve Road, Artarmon NSW 2064, Australia

National Library of Australia
Cataloguing-in-Publication data:

Hawe, Penelope
Evaluating health promotion, a health worker's guide
Bibliography
Includes index
ISBN 0 86433 067 7

1. Health promotion — Evaluation
2. Health education — Evaluation. I Degeling
Deirdre E. II. Hall, Jane. III Title
613.07

Printed and bound in Australia

Foreword

All too frequently, health promotion programmes have been established on the basis of limited research, and implemented with little or no evaluation. As a consequence, many programmes have been established with poorly conceived and unrealistic objectives, and with no effective mechanism for management, quality control or monitoring. Such programmes are often doomed to failure, and even where 'successful', have not been capable of yielding supportive evidence to ensure their continued existence.

Evaluating Health Promotion can help change this rather gloomy picture. There can be no doubt that better quality evaluation in health promotion will lead to better interventions. Better evaluation will also contribute to a wider acknowledgement of the contribution of health promotion to improving the public health. This book is deceptively simple in design and layout, and yet provides a comprehensive and common-sense guide to the evaluation process, using well chosen examples to illustrate the key steps along the way. Chapter by chapter the book shows how a more systematic approach to evaluation will impose greater discipline to the tasks of needs assessment and programme planning. It shows how well conceived evaluation can provide project managers with useful feedback on programme implementation and development as the intervention unfolds. The book also illustrates the range of evaluation methods to provide evidence of the impact and outcome of health promotion programmes— a complex but essential part of the evaluation process for practitioners, managers and funders alike.

Evaluating Health Promotion has been thoughtfully assembled by authors who have obvious practical experience in programme management and delivery. It deals with the key issues in a systematic way, providing the reader with a 'user-friendly' guide to both the science and art of evaluation in health promotion. The book's greatest strength lies in the fact that it has been written by practitioners for practitioners in such a way as to build skills and inspire confidence for good quality evaluation. To ensure a sound, secure and substantial improvement in health promotion practice in the 1990's will require better quality evaluation which is more fully integrated with the planning and implementation of programmes. This book will make a substantial contribution to that process.

Don Nutbeam
Professor of Public Health
University of Sydney

Contents

Part 2

PROGRAMME EVALUATION: THE SKILLS YOU NEED

Acknowledgements

We are grateful to Janene Waters for assistance with the chapters on focus groups and literature review. Christine Ewan advised us on instructional design. Christopher Rissel undertook part of the initial literature research and planning.

Special thanks to Jason Grossman for his work on the bibliography, research assistance and for his valuable comments on the text.

Alan Owen, Louise Rowling and Margaret Hamilton carefully reviewed an earlier draft and provided excellent criticism and useful suggestions.

Professor Stephen Leeder and the staff of the Department of Community Medicine at Westmead Hospital provided encouragement, inspiration, advice and support.

We wish to thank the Commonwealth Department of Community Services and Health for a National Health Promotion Programme Grant and Health Departments in the states of South Australia, Victoria, Tasmania, Queensland and New South Wales for help in organising the workshop series which allowed us to develop and test the materials presented in this book.

In particular, we are indebted to the hundreds of health workers who became involved in the project. Their experience of health promotion evaluation and their enthusiasm for it demanded that a book such as this be written.

About This Book

This book is written for people whose main responsibility is to design and run health promotion programmes, not research them. The main focus therefore is on those evaluation tasks which can be usefully undertaken by programme staff, in an attempt to strengthen the contribution to health promotion evaluation made by field workers as distinct from those advances made by people engaged in full-time research.

In putting together material and examples we have drawn on the ideas and experience of many health workers in community and hospital settings in this country. Health promotion is interpreted and practised in many different ways. We do not attempt to reconcile different viewpoints in health promotion. We attempt to offer an evaluation approach which encourages all practitioners to reflect on their own way of thinking and at the same time collects evidence about programme performance which stands up to outside scrutiny. Evaluation is a powerful tool and in promoting health promotion evaluation we have tried to ground it as a skill firmly belonging in the hands of the health workers and their communities involved in intervention development. Evaluation is not just as an 'add on' technical activity.

In the approach we present, the first step in evaluation is to have the right programme. This is why the topics covered in the early chapters are on needs assessment and programme planning. Showing that a poorly targetted or poorly designed programme does not work is a waste of energy. Time is better spent in designing a good programme than in rushing out to evaluate what you suspect might be a bad one. Later chapters outline methods for assessing programme activity and programme effects. The second half of the book is devoted to particular skills in evaluation, including how to access and work with other people with special skills to contribute.

PART 1

Programme Evaluation:
What you need to know

Chapter 1

THINKING ABOUT EVALUATION BEFORE YOU START YOUR PROGRAMME

A Commitment to Good Practice

Improving health. Preventing illness. Preventing premature mortality. Improving quality of life. Strengthening the capacity to cope. How often have we heard these phrases in recent years? It would be easy to think that the need to address these issues is new, but it is not new. People who have been closely involved with health promotion have been concerned with these issues for many years. What is new is the increasing government interest in health promotion as a result of the ageing of the population, rising health care costs, the widening social class gradient in health and pressure from health lobby groups. Health promotion is under new scrutiny. People who practise health promotion are now being asked to show what they have to offer.

Health promotion is defined by Green and Anderson as:

> *Any combination of health education and related organisational, economic and environmental supports for behaviour of individuals, groups or communities conducive to health.*[1]

The Ottawa Charter for health promotion lays a different emphasis:

> *Health promotion is the process of enabling people to increase control over, and to improve, their health. To reach a state of complete physical, mental and social well being an individual or group must be able to identify and realise aspirations, to satisfy needs and to change or cope with the environment.*[2]

In practice, a range of different interventions is called health promotion and some examples are given in Table 1.

People who practise health promotion work in a variety of settings

3

Table 1. *Some examples of health promotion.*

	Example
Teaching patients skills to promote self-care and self-management of their illness.	asthma education, medication education
Teaching teachers about common childhood disorders, such as epilepsy and asthma to promote better management in the classroom	teacher education
Raising community awareness about health hazards and health risks	mass media campaigns
Setting up self-help groups among people who share a common life situation, illness or condition to promote information sharing, mutual help and social support	new parent group grief and loss groups cancer support groups
Setting up social networks among at-risk populations such as the elderly, new migrant groups, residents of new housing estates to promote information sharing and social support	neighbourhood contact schemes, mobile information and activity vans
Helping local residents, groups and agencies to develop the skills and resources to lobby on issues to improve the health and quality of life in the community, such as child care services, better health services, better public transport, more school crossings, less environmental pollution	community development, community organisation, community action
Setting up mechanisms to promote community involvement in planning and decision making which affects the community's health and quality of life	community management of services and organisations, community participation
Alerting individuals to their personal risk of developing illness and advising how to make changes to their style of life	cholesterol screening, risk factor assessment and counselling
Group programmes to change health habits and style of life in order to reduce health risk	weight control groups, smoking cessation groups
Legislative change to reduce health risks	seat belt laws, school immunization laws

such as schools, hospitals, community health centres, community agencies, local government and worksites.

Some people work exclusively in one field, such as in patient education or in community development. The emphasis of some programmes is on self-help or individual self-management for health. The emphasis of other programmes is on collective action for community health. With some interventions, changes in health or actions taken for health are made anonymously and individually, like responding to a media 'quit smoking' message. With other interventions the target group's involvement is more visible and central to the strategy of the programme, such as helping a local community to collect data about health needs and develop ways to address these needs.

Few people would argue with the intention of health promotion. Many health workers define health promotion as part of their role, even those in traditional curative settings. Many different types of professions and agencies are eager to undertake health promotion. The question is whether they have a commitment to do it well.

Good practice in health promotion is not instinctive. Some large-scale community demonstration projects have failed to achieve their goals.[3] It has been claimed that some health promotion programmes have made problems worse, such as interventions which increased experimental drug taking among adolescents[4] and increased motor vehicle accidents.[5,6] Enthusiastic efforts to mass-produce health information for the public have resulted in publications which a large proportion of the population cannot understand.[7] Some evidence suggests that health education campaigns have actually widened the information gap between the more and less well educated groups.[8] Even the self-help movement has come under criticism because of its potential to encourage people to become involved in cathartic exchanges and discussions about the nature of the problem or the condition rather than focusing attention on external factors that may be the cause of the problem and where the real resolution to the problem may lie.[9]

A commitment to good health promotion practice means a commitment to planning and evaluation of programmes. Planning, to take in the needs of the target group and the best of current knowledge as to how to meet these needs. Evaluation, to find out the effect of the programme, who has benefitted and who has not.

As you will see from the size of this book, a commitment to planning and evaluation in health promotion is not something to be taken lightly. It means acknowledging your responsibility to deliver the best intervention you can within your resources. It means that your programme will build on what others have learned and that you will conduct your programme and your evaluation in a way that others will learn from it. Although there is enormous diversity in the approaches to health promotion which people prefer, people who practise health promotion should be united in their commitment to do it well. Further, we are now working in a climate in which we will be judged not on our intentions, or our philosophies or our enthusiasm, but on what difference we make to people's lives. The people who sit in judgement are not only the governments, administrators or communities we serve, the judges are also ourselves and the confidence with which we say that we are making a true contribution.

What Does 'Evaluation' Mean?

Trouble? A lot of money? A waste of time? In some ways health workers could be justified in being a little dubious about evaluation because in the health and social services it has a long history of abuse. People talk about evaluating programmes to delay making decisions about them. They evaluate programmes as the lead-up to cutting back on the programme. Or they evaluate only the bad aspects of a good programme or only the good aspects of a bad programme.[10] They may make up their mind about a programme and then collect only data that supports their point of view. In health promotion we also run the risk of smothering an exciting new programme, by weighing it down with an evaluation research protocol that is insensitive to what the programme is about.

In the first instance, evaluation requires sorting through some of these problems and acknowledging that in health services and in health promotion, evaluation research is a rational process trying to carve out a niche in a political environment.

Suchman's definition of evaluation illustrates an important point:

> *Evaluation is the process by which we judge the worth or value of something.*[10]

Notice the word 'value' in the word 'evaluation'. Evaluation is a judgement about something. How you judge it depends on expectations, past experience, what you think is important, what you think is not important. This affects how the evaluation is conducted, whose interests it serves and what methods you use. Different groups may evaluate programmes differently with different outcomes and conclusions. For example, the Australian Consumers' Association has recently conducted an evaluation of the major clinics involved in in-vitro fertilization (IVF) and assessed the extent of written information and whether it adequately presents the risks, inconveniences and possible complications. Their conclusion was that most IVF couples are failing to receive full, written and unbiased information, which makes it difficult for couples to make informed decisions about their participation in the programme.[11] By contrast, the scientists involved with IVF in their reported evaluations focus on such issues as cost effectiveness.[12] Neither evaluation is 'right' and both groups would probably be interested in the data produced by both investigations, but given the choice, each group decided to conduct its evaluation differently, focusing on the issues of most interest to it.

There are two ways to make an evaluation. You can just make a judgement about a programme. You can say 'It's a good programme'. Another way is to collect some data about the programme and use this to make your judgement. This might include opinion data but also might include data on the changes the programme has made, who the programme has reached, the long-term effects and so on. Once you start doing research to help you make an evaluation this is termed 'evaluative research',[10] though in everyday language health workers often use the word 'evaluation' when what they are strictly referring to is 'evaluative research' or 'evaluation research.'

Evaluation (evaluative research) is not the same as ordinary research. This is because evaluation involves more than just making observations and collecting data. Evaluation involves two processes— (1) observation and measurement and then (2) comparison of what you observe with some criterion or standard of what you (or the group you represent) would consider an indication of good performance.[13]

For example, after you run a fitness campaign you can collect all the data you like about the number of people in your local area who say that they exercise regularly, which is the research part, but this won't tell you that your campaign has been successful. To do this you must already have in mind a figure about the proportion of the population who should be exercising. This might correspond to a national health goal or target.

So, programme evaluation usually involves observing and collecting measures about how a programme operates and the effects it appears to be having and comparing this to a pre-set standard or yardstick. Before you set out to collect data you should know the standard or criterion by which you will judge your results. For example, a baby health nurse may state that preparation for parenthood classes will be considered successful in reaching the target group if 80% of all pregnant women registering at the hospital for their confinements attend the classes. A psychologist running self-esteem classes for adolescents may state that the programme will be considered a success (and will be duplicated in other schools) if 65% or more students show a marked improvement as indicated by a particular scale or inventory.

Later we will discuss where these standards or yardsticks for performance come from. The reason why the criteria by which you will judge the programme should be specified first is that after you go out and collect a whole lot of data about the programme, it will be tempting to call any level of improvement or change a success! Also, setting out very clearly the process by which the programme will be judged does not eliminate the values which influence how the judgement about the programme is made, but it at least holds them up to public scrutiny.

Approaches to Evaluation: Qualitative and Quantitative

Evaluation is not an absolute science. There is no right or wrong way to evaluate a programme because, as illustrated earlier, people have different ideas about what sort of information about a programme is important. If the main emphasis of the evaluation is on participant satisfaction, for example, the evaluation method will differ from that when the main emphasis of the evaluation is an assessment of costs and benefits. The issue here is to design an evaluation appropriate to the type of information needed about the programme.

Often a distinction is made between qualitative and quantitative approaches to evaluation. Qualitative methods attempt to determine the meaning and experience of the programme for the people involved and to interpret effects that may be observed. The approach is unstructured and the evaluator is led by what people say about the programme. Quantitative methods on the other hand attempt to measure and 'score' changes occurring as a result of the programme and measures may be made systematically on each participant using instruments preselected to detect the sort of changes the evaluator expects to see. Quantitative approaches usually gain less-detailed information from a larger number of participants than qualitative methods, but have the advantage that they are considered to be better suited to developing the type of evaluation designs set up to test the extent to which a programme causes changes in health status, health behaviour, knowledge and so on.

Again no single approach is 'right' and the appropriate choice of qualitative and quantitative methods depends very much on: (1) the sort of question your evaluation is trying to answer and the type of data required by the people who will use your evaluation to make decisions about the future of the programme; and (2) the stage of the programme's development. Many evaluations combine qualitative and quantitative approaches.

Let's say that you have been involved in running a new programme to help equip community residents in the skills required for effective participation in area health planning and administration (how to access local databases, meeting procedures, techniques for conflict resolution and so on). Your evaluation is trying to find out if participants feel that they have benefitted from your programme and where they feel there may be gaps in the programme. This is the sort of situation well suited to a qualitative investigation.

Let's consider another situation, say a school-based smoking prevention programme. To find out if the programme is effective, it is unlikely that the decision makers funding this sort of programme would be convinced just by the results of interviews with students and teachers about what they thought of the programme. They may want you to find out what proportion of children were prevented from taking up smoking by the programme. This is suited to a quantitative evaluation approach.

The stage of a programme's development is critical to the type of approach you take in evaluation. For example, in the early stages of a very new programme, you may be uncertain as to what the effects are likely to be. Logically, you have to know what you are looking for before you can work out how to quantify it. So a quantitative approach may follow an initial qualitative investigation.

Finally, you might also consider the reality that some funding authorities are more familiar with certain approaches. A pragmatic argument for quantitative approaches in health promotion evaluation would be simply that decision makers who are currently funding programmes in curative medicine will be more likely to divert funds into prevention if they are presented with the same sort of evidence for programme effectiveness in prevention as they are used to getting from advocates of, say, coronary care units or other curative services. This sort of evidence is usually quantitative and generated from experimental or quasi-experimental designs.

However, this is not an invitation to brutalize your programme to fit a particular evaluation mould if this is not appropriate. There are many occasions when an experimental approach is neither feasible nor desirable.[14] Further, you may not always be able to find a measure to quantify the effects of your programme which adequately captures the magic or essence of what occurs. Evaluation techniques frequently lag behind innovation in programme development and there is a responsibility to sensitize and educate decision makers and funding authorities about appropriate evidence for programme effectiveness.

How Much Work is Involved in Evaluation? Can the Tasks Be Shared?

Consider the following case study.

> A baby health nurse and preschool social worker design a special programme to provide health information and social support to pregnant adolescents. They are concerned not only about the young woman's health and feelings about herself and her situation, but also about the health of the baby and the family environment about to be created by that child and mother.
>
> Let's suppose that the programme involves maternal and child health staff in home visits and weekly education and discussion sessions for periods up to 6 months before the birth and 12 months afterwards. A group of 18 young women is involved in the first programme. To evaluate the effect of the programme, data are collected from medical records, infant welfare records and from interviews with the adolescents involved. Results indicate that the women participating in the programme subsequently do not have birth complications and babies with birth weights lower or worse than the hospital average. Immunization rates and attendance at well baby clinics are better than expected for mothers of that age. The young mothers involved in the programme report feeling well

supported and comfortable in their new role. But in spite of this, the Regional Director of Health is not prepared to accept the recommendation from this evaluation that resources be allocated to duplicate this programme in other areas. Why?

It is possible to argue that the young women in this programme would have achieved good perinatal outcomes and good immunization rates anyway. It may be that the young women who volunteer to be involved in these sorts of programmes are at lower risk than the shy and isolated young women who drop out or who choose not to be involved in the first place. Without the opportunity to observe a comparison group, that is a group of similar adolescents who didn't receive the programme, it is not possible to conclude that it was the programme that produced the results we saw.

Further, the numbers involved in this evaluation were quite small. Statistical theory tells us that to detect an effect of the programme, say, in improving children's vaccination rates from 60% to 80%, you would need to have 108 women in the programme group and another 108 women in the comparison group. With fewer numbers an important difference between the groups may not be detected. Now, a baby health nurse and a social worker have other responsibilities and probably not the time to conduct an evaluation on the scale being outlined. But by bringing this programme to the attention of administrators and decision makers with inadequate evidence to support the recommendations, it makes it easy for administrators to dismiss the programme entirely. A potentially good programme may be lost.

What would have been a better way to tackle the evaluation of this programme? We have said that to demonstrate success in terms of perinatal morbidity, attendance at well baby clinics or subsequent vaccination rates, a major study is needed. What may make administrators devote the extra resources required for such a study? What sort of information can be collected to demonstrate that such an undertaking is worthwhile?

Before a large-scale study is undertaken to investigate programme effects, some other evaluation work should be completed. Firstly you need information to assure you that your programme is reaching the right group, the at-risk pregnant adolescents, and that they are truly at risk of poor perinatal outcome. When the programme is operating you need information to assure you that the programme is running the way it should, that attendance is high, that the group leaders communicate well, that participants seem to get a lot from coming along, that other programme staff perform their roles competently and so on. Without knowing that the programme is operating well and getting to the right groups you would not expect it to make a difference to maternal and infant health anyway. Data about programme reach and programme implementation should be collected first. These data could then be

Table 2. *Suggested sharing of evaluation tasks in health promotion programme evaluation.*

Evaluation task	Person responsible
Finding out if the programme is reaching the target group	
Observing programme operations to see if the programme is being implemented properly	
Assessing participant's satisfaction with the programme	Programme staff
Assessing programme quality	
Making a preliminary assessment of programme effects	
Assessing the short-term effects and determining if they are really caused by the programme	Evaluation research staff
Assessing longer-term effects and determining if they are really caused by the programme	

used to support a submission for further funds to collect data about the programme's effects. The reason why you need more resources to continue your evaluation is because of the point mentioned earlier. When an investigation of programme effects involves making inferences about causality, it frequently involves large sample sizes and measuring changes in a comparison group. This means collecting data from more people than those usually serviced by the programme so more staff are needed.

Table 2 illustrates some sharing in evaluation tasks that could take place between programme staff, the people who design and run the programme and evaluation research staff, who are brought in when preliminary work indicates that an investigation of programme effects is worth doing.

The suggested sharing of responsibilities between programme staff is defined by a number of parameters. First of all the tasks listed for the programme staff logically come first. By completing these tasks, the programme staff ensure that the evaluation of programme effects is not going to happen prematurely, that is, before the programme is likely to have an effect. Should programme staff find that the programme is functioning less well than expected they can take steps to improve the programme before the assessment of programme effects. The tasks listed for programme staff are also those which do not require a lot of time and resources. By contrast, the tasks listed for evaluation research staff may involve collecting a lot of information from large groups over a long period. For example, in the evaluation of a patient education programme in which one of us was recently involved, when the evaluation was assessing only before-programme and after-programme changes in knowledge among participants, the programme budget was $8000 per year. When the evaluation set out to determine if the programme was causing changes in behaviour and whether these changes were sustained over a three-month period, the programme budget rose to $32 000 per year, to pay for interviewers making assessments on an experimental and control group, once before the programme and twice afterwards.

The sharing of responsibilities between programme staff and evaluation research staff also attempts to make the best of the input from internal and external evaluators. For example, programme staff on the whole are probably better able than outside people to observe the programme operations closely—communicating effectively with the target group, collecting data unobtrusively and sensitively and feeding information back in a manner which encourages improvement in the programme. On the other hand, when it comes to assessing programme effects it may be hard for programme staff to be objective and impossible for them to cooperate in the type of evaluation design where the interviewers are not aware of the identity of the experimental group (the people who receive the programme) and the control group (similar people who do not receive the programme).

By splitting up responsibilities in this way we do not wish to imply that programme staff and evaluation research staff have to keep strictly to these roles all the time. In fact, a lot would be gained by both parties if staff had the opportunity on occasions to participate at each end. The purpose of the role proposal is to make sure that (1) programme staff do not get pressured into those evaluation tasks which they are not usually equipped to undertake and (2) evaluation research staff do not undertake some types of evaluation tasks until certain other evaluation work has been completed. These recommendations are to avoid two main problems in programme evaluation—(1) having inadequate evidence on which to base claims about programme effectiveness (like the baby health nurse and preschool social worker in our earlier example) and (2) evaluating a programme prematurely, before it is functioning optimally and likely to be having an effect.

It is not unusual to suggest that all the evaluation tasks necessary in health promotion cannot be undertaken by the people who design and conduct the programmes. After all, we do not expect a doctor prescribing a particular medication to have done the clinical trial that demonstrated its superiority to another drug. However, in health promotion the notion has unfortunately developed that programme staff have to show that their programmes increase Pap smears, improve immunisation rates, prevent unnecessary hospital admissions and so on. We agree that this work must be done, but it is not possible to do so within a programme budget. When it is time to assess programme effects, a major evaluative study is involved. Additional resources will be required and this is likely to mean a separate evaluation budget and additional staff. Programme staff could elect to undertake the evaluation tasks involved in the major study, but they would have to find other people to run the programme for them. Either way, additional resources would be needed.

Does it Still Sound Daunting?
Why Bother with Evaluation?

By sharing the evaluation responsibilities with other staff the evaluation tasks for the people who also run the programmes may now be more 'do-able'. But maybe you still have doubts as to why all this is necessary.

We have stated that one reason to evaluate is to make sure that at a minimum your programme is not making the problem worse. In a commitment to good practice, you should be evaluating to ensure that your programme is making a useful contribution. Evaluation also provides rewarding feedback about progress. Maybe if health workers received this feedback more often there would be less tendency to burnout. Many health workers in the public sector would rather see more clients, write up case notes or go to another meeting than take the time to write up the conclusions from the experience of conducting an evaluation of their programmes. However, by not taking this step, people may cheat themselves of some recognition and support which they could gain for their activities. In health promotion, although the highest profile seems to go to those large-scale, often academically linked programmes in, say, smoking cessation or heart disease prevention,[15-17] surveys have shown that the bulk of health promotion programmes is smaller-scale interventions conducted by health workers in community health centres and hospitals.[18] If health workers in these settings could be encouraged to evaluate and document their work, the role of health promotion at this level would be reinforced and made more obvious to funding authorities.

Evaluation of health promotion also contributes to theory building in health promotion. Changing people's health and quality of life is not easily done. It is based on an understanding of the motivations, predispositions, reinforcements, values, beliefs, social, financial, legal and political processes that shape our lives. A programme that can bring about an improvement for people must be communicated to others so that more people can benefit. A programme which fails to bring about an improvement must be carefully reconsidered, as the assumptions and theory behind the programme may be incorrect. Either way, with success or failure, the experience of conducting the evaluation brings benefit to the field.

This is a critical point. Many health workers are nervous of the terms 'success' or 'failure' in relation to health promotion programmes, as if in some way programme performance is tied directly to their own professional self-esteem. To avoid failure they avoid evaluation. This is unfortunate. Health promotion is a dynamic and rapidly changing field. At any one time many of the current initiatives may turn out to be those that fail to produce the intended results. There is no shame in this. It is simply a reflection of the state of a developing field. It provides incentive for shifts in thinking and radical new approaches. A lot of what happens will be unexpected. Stigma should not be attached to programmes that fail, only to those programmes that fail to learn from these experiences or to those programmes that fail to evaluate.

References

1. Green LW, Anderson CL. *Community Health.* St. Louis: Times Mirror/Mosby College Publishing, 1986;516.
2. Ottawa Charter for Health Promotion. International Conference on Health Promotion 17–21 November 1986. Ottawa: World Health Organisation.
3. Rose G, Tunstall-Pedoe HD, Heller RF. UK heart disease prevention project: Incidence and mortality results. *Lancet* 1983;1:1062–1065.
4. Berberian RM. The relationship between drug education programmes in the greater New Haven schools and changes in drug use and drug related beliefs and perceptions. *Health Education Monographs* 1976;4:327–376.
5. Robertson LS, Zador PL. Driver education and crash involvement of teenaged drivers. *American Journal of Public Health* 1978;68:959–965.
6. Robertson LS. Crash involvement of teenaged drivers when education is eliminated from high school. *American Journal of Public Health* 1980;70:599–603.
7. Bauman AE, Smith NA, Braithwaite C, Free A, Saunders A. Asthma information: can it be understood? *Health Education Research* 1989;4(3):377–382
8. Ettema JS, Brown JW, Leupker RV. Knowledge gap effects in a health information campaign. *Public Opinion Quarterly* 1983;47:516–527.
9. Sidel VW, Sidel R. Beyond Coping. *Social Policy* 1976;–Sept-Oct:67–69.
10. Suchman EA. *Evaluative Research.* New York: Russell Sage Foundation, 1967.
11. Australian Consumers' Association. IVF A plea for honesty. *Choice* 1989;30(10):17–25.
12. Jansen R. The clinical impact of invitro fertilisation Part 2 Regulation, money and research. *Medical Journal of Australia* 1987;146:362–366.
13. Deniston OL. Whither evaluation—whither utilisation. *Evaluation and Program Planning* 1980;3:91–94.
14. Smith NL. The feasability and desirability of experimental methods in evaluation. *Evaluation and Program Planning* 1980;3:251–256.
15. Pierce JP, Dwyer T, Frape G, Chapman S, Chamberlin A, Burke N. Evaluation of the Sydney 'Quit. For Life' anti smoking campaign. Part 1 Achievement of intermediate goals. *Medical Journal of Australia* 1986;144:341–344.

16. Dwyer T, Pierce JP, Hannam CD, Burke N. Evaluation of the changes in smoking prevalence. *Medical Journal of Australia* 1986;144:344–347.
17. Farquar J, Macoby N, Wood PD, Alexander JK, Breitrose H, Brown BW Jnr, Haskell WL, McAlister AL, Meyer A, Nash JD, Stern MP. Community education for cardiovascular health. *Lancet* 1977;1:1191–1195.
18. Hall J, Hawe P, Degeling D, Moore A. *A cross sectional survey of health promotion programmes in NSW in 1983*. Department of Community Medicine Monograph. Sydney: Westmead Hospital, 1984.

Further Reading

Braverman MT, ed. *Evaluating Health Promotion Programs*. San Francisco: Jossey Bass, 1989.
Ross HS, Mico PR. *Theory and Practice in Health Education*. Palo Alto California: Mayfield Publishing Company, 1980.

Chapter 2

NEEDS ASSESSMENT: WHAT ISSUE SHOULD YOUR PROGRAMME ADDRESS?

OBJECTIVES

At the end of this chapter you should be able to:

1. Define what is meant by 'need'.
2. List and describe the different types of need.
3. Facilitate community involvement in the identification of health needs and priorities.
4. Locate and interpret health status data and sociodemographic data for your area or population group.
5. Identify the criteria you will use to select a priority health problem.
6. Identify and collect additional data to gain more insight into the health problem you have chosen.
7. Analyse factors contributing to the health problem in your community and sort these into an order to help you determine the focal points for intervention (risk markers, risk factors and factors contributing to the risk factors).

Consider all the different health promotion programmes your agency is involved with. Why did they get started? Do programmes reflect the needs of the community or just the talents of the staff? Do programmes simply reflect tradition? What groups are served by the programmes? What groups miss out?

In this chapter we will be looking at how you identify health needs and determine priority among them. We will address the sort of data needed to describe the characteristics of your target group and also the sort of data needed about factors that might contribute to the health problem which may be the focus of your intervention. Finally we discuss some of the difficult issues associated with needs assessment such as the resolution of conflict between the priority interests of different groups.

What do we Mean by 'Need'?

Activity

Take a few minutes to think about what you are actually referring to when you use the word 'need' or 'needs assessment'.

Feedback

It's difficult, isn't it? 'Need' in health promotion is something we all seem to refer to without specifying exactly what we mean. One definition for 'need' has been offered by Denton:

> *. . . a need is defined as a state, situation or condition in the community which by its presence or absence reduces, limits or prevents normative function.* [1]

In other words, satisfaction of needs corresponds to living and functioning according to the standard or norm desirable in the community. Health needs are understood as being those states, conditions or factors in the community which, if absent, prevent people from achieving the optimum of physical, mental and social well-being. This would include such things as provision of health services and health information, a safe physical environment, productive work and/or activity and a network of emotionally supportive and stimulating relationships. Using this sort of definition, disease states, such as arthritis, and risk factors, such as smoking, also come under the definition of need as we believe that having this condition or this behaviour ultimately will limit the individual's functional capacity. You can also see in this definition that need is a relative concept. It depends on our view of how things should be and clearly, people will not always agree with each other or even think the same way in 5 or 10 years' time.

It is important to note that when they are talking about need sometimes people interchange the concept of the need state or condition they are describing with what they consider the solution to the problem to be. For example, instead of saying that the problem or health need is poor oral health, they might say that the need is for more dentists. Instead of saying that a high proportion of adolescents are obese, they might say that school-based weight control programmes are needed.

There is a danger in this sort of confusion. What we might see as the satisfactory solution for a problem changes across time and is nearly always influenced by different values, experiences, interests and expectations. For example, in recent years many women have felt alienated by health care providers and have felt unsatisfied with the care given to them, but there has been debate about whether this can be solved by setting up special women's health centres or instead running training programmes for general practitioners to better sensitize them to women's health needs.

In the first instance, it is better to direct people to a careful description and understanding of the problem and how it is being experienced and postpone argument about what might be the answer to the problem, as this may lead to the problem itself being obscured. The purpose of needs assessment is to do just this. After the problems have been understood, and one has been chosen as the first priority, a range of possible solutions might be put forward. This is a separate step in the process of programme planning and evaluation which we deal with in the next chapter.

Types of Need

You can see that the concept of need leaves a lot of room for interpretation about how a need would be recognized and expressed. Bradshaw[2] has suggested that there are four dimensions or different types of need and each is identified using different methods. By tapping into each dimension of need you will increase your chance of constructing a comprehensive picture of community problems. You may also realize that many different organizations, professionals and interest groups limit themselves to just one dimension!

Normative need
Normative need has come to refer to what expert opinion defines as need. For example, the National Health and Medical Research Council has a recommendation that all children aged 12 to 15 months be vaccinated against measles. If a survey showed that many children were unimmunized, then this would indicate a health need.

Normative need governs a great deal of health planning. Be aware, however, that normative standards often differ between different groups of experts and change over time. For example, in 1986 the National Heart Foundation considered serum cholesterol levels of 6.5 mmol/L as requiring medical intervention, but then lowered the critical point to 5.6 mmol/L and currently recommends that any level above 5.2 mmol/L warrants intervention.

Expressed need
Expressed need refers to what you can infer about the health need of a community by observation of their use of services. Heavy booking at

a birthing centre, for example, expresses people's preference for alternative obstetric services to traditional hospital care. Long waiting lists at child guidance clinics may indicate that there are more problems in the psychological and social adjustment of children than can be catered for by existing services.

However, expressed need can be misinterpreted. Long waiting lists at a health service may be more an indicator that the service is slow or inefficient than it may indicate something about the size of the group waiting to be treated. Also, if you only make inferences about community needs from a community's use of services then you will completely miss out on an understanding of those needs for which no service is currently provided. A community with no child care services is not necessarily a community with no need for child care.

Comparative need

Comparative need is need derived from examining the services provided in one area to one population and using this as the basis to determine the sort of services needed in another area with a similar population. We see this when new hospitals are built in outer suburban areas because these areas have fewer hospital beds per person than inner-city areas. This way of deriving need on the basis of comparison of per capita levels of service provision is very common. We hear people referring to areas which are 'less well served' with respect to urological services, speech therapy and so on.

There is a problem in relying on need derived by comparison. This problem is the underlying assumption that the level of service provision in the reference area is appropriate in the first place. The level of service provision may in fact be a reflection of overservicing by service providers rather than an indication of true need for the service by health consumers. In other words, the reliance on comparative need as a basis of health planning leads to similarity in patterns of service provision and this does not necessarily reflect adequate or appropriate service provision.

Felt need

Felt need is what people in your community say they want or what they think are the problems that need addressing. Common methods of assessing felt needs are household opinion surveys, phone-ins, public meetings, calling for submissions and so on.

There are three things to note when determining felt needs. The first is one that was mentioned earlier and that is the tendency for people to express the need in terms of its solution rather than stating the need itself (for example, 'more nursing home beds'). The second thing to be aware of is who the person espousing the need represents. Are they speaking for themselves? Are they making inferences about the needs of others and who are they? The third thing to look out for is how you interpret people reporting that they are satisfied with services. It is very common, for example, for some people passively to accept what other people might consider a poor situation or level of care. So when people say they are satisfied with something you have to take into account their expectations as well as the nature of the service that was provided.

Activity

The following are examples of different types of need. Can you identify which is normative, expressed, comparative and felt need?

1. A waiting list for orthopaedic surgery used as an argument to support appointment of another surgeon.
2. A residents' petition for a dental service.
3. Data from the Health Department's recent survey showing that few adolescents practise safe sex, used to support a health promotion funding application.
4. A commissioned report from a private consultancy firm that indicates that the region has fewer psychiatric beds than the rest of the state and recommends that a psychiatric unit be established.

Feedback

1. Expressed need.
2. Felt need; note that it focusses on a solution to the problem.
3. Normative need—experts' knowledge about the transmission of AIDS and its importance is illustrated in this need.
4. Comparative need.

The reason why it is important for you to be able to classify and recognize different types of need when they are presented to you is because this will immediately help you to be aware of the strengths and weaknesses in each type of approach. It should be stressed again that need is a relative concept and different groups will value different types of needs differently. There will be debate over what constitutes adequate or poor care, or satisfactory or unsatisfactory service provision. When you ask people to nominate what the needs are, you will nearly always come up with a never-ending list, so it will be necessary to bring in a concept of most important or less important needs, and priority order.

Some professional groups also use the terms differently. Health economists, for example, use 'need' to refer to a concept more closely associated with what we have described as normative need. They use the term 'want' to refer to felt needs and 'demand' to refer to expressed needs. This is why you need to be clear about what people mean when they use different terms, what evidence they may have and what assumptions they may have made when they talk about needs.

Steps in Needs Assessment

Needs assessments are conducted in order to get a comprehensive picture of the health problems in the community and thus guide the choices about the sorts of health interventions that should be planned and mounted. Data sources and opinions are canvassed widely to help make the right choices. To make the right choices, you also need to be very aware of the criteria used to make the decision.

Needs assessment does not have to be a tiresome, passive, data burdensome process. Indeed, writers in this field have urged health educators to adopt the attitude that needs assessment on a local level can be part of the intervention process itself and the beginning of active community interest and involvement.[3] In this way the skills involved in needs assessment cover not only data collection, analysis and interpretation but also community consultation, communication skills and consensus building skills.[3]

However, as you will see shortly, your role in needs assessment depends very much on your position in your organization, your health promotion philosophy, the mission of your agency and the extent to which the direction of your planning in health promotion has been left open. In many cases health policy makers and planners may have already identified the major health problems that should be tackled. This would correspond, for example, to our national health goals. Your job may simply be to initiate action on the local level. In other circumstances, you may be in a position to explore local concerns which may or may not correspond with the national interest. Even in relation to national health goals, though, there is a view that communities must gather data and view their own situation and translate goals into something achievable on the local level for there to be an impetus for action.[4]

Needs assessment can be divided into two main stages according to the purpose of the data collection at each stage. The steps will embrace all dimensions of need (normative, expressed, felt and comparative) and the mix of these is up to you according to the options available to you.

The two stages in needs assessment are as follows:

Stage I Identifying the priority health problem
Steps 1–4.
> The purpose is to collect data and canvass a range of opinions to determine among these a priority health problem. The magnitude

of the problem should be clearly specified along with details about the target group experiencing the problem.

Stage II   Analysis of the health problem
Steps 5–9.

The purpose is to collect additional data about the factors that are contributing to the health problem as these may become the focus of subsequent intervention. These factors are sorted into classes which help explain why the problem is occurring and being maintained.

Your starting point in needs assessment depends on the sort of brief you have been given in your job or agency and the role you have adopted as a health worker. If you have been appointed to work in the area of cardiovascular risk reduction or community nutrition or drug abuse prevention, policy makers and planners have reached the decision made at the end of Stage I in needs assessment. That is, the health problem and perhaps also the target group have already been selected. In this case you may decide to proceed directly to the beginning of Stage II of needs assessment to collect the sort of data you will need to plan your intervention.

Alternatively, you may be in a position to start from the beginning. The community's needs have not been determined and put into priority order. Data about community risk for different health problems may not be known. In this case your starting point in needs assessment is Step 1 in Stage I, bearing in mind that some work in Stage I may have been covered by policy makers and planners and you should be aware of this.

Each of these steps will now be described in turn. They are presented as a linear sequence simply to illustrate the logic of the process. You may find, however, depending on the community you are working with, the purpose of your needs assessment and the work that might have gone on beforehand, that you spend more or less time in each of these steps.

Stage I   Identifying the Priority Health Problem
Step 1   Consultation

The first step involves going out and talking to some of the people living and working in the community to get a feel for the sorts of issues and areas that are likely to be important. What seem to be the main health problems or concerns? What do health workers think? What groups are experiencing these problems? Go to health agencies, community organizations, volunteer networks, local doctors, midwives, researchers, ethnic organizations, teachers and so on. Talk to a range of people to get an understanding of the breadth and depth of point of view. Maybe people are worried about illegal drug use, adolescent pregnancy, or social isolation and depression in the elderly. You should develop an understanding of the sorts of issues you might then follow up more systematically. Remember that people will be expressing points of view and experience of different types of need and that there is likely to be conflict and disagreement. You should also use this opportunity to seek out the results of any surveys or community research that may have been carried out previously.

Step 2   Data collection

Now you should pause and take stock a little. There are some existing sources of data that could be useful. These pertain to descriptions of the make-up or composition of your population (to assist in making inferences about the sorts of needs that may emerge) and data directly concerning the population's health and health service use. After review of these data you will be in a position to make decisions about any additional data which you may need to collect yourself.

Activity
Where would you go to find out more about the community's characteristics and also its health problems? What type of data would you hope to gather?

Feedback
Let's start with the community's characteristics. The Australian Bureau of Statistics (ABS) and various other state and national authorities collect a great deal of data that can be used in health promotion planning. In some cases you might be able to get data quite specific to your local area (for example, the size of a district covered by a single collector for the census). State and regional offices of the health department may have already compiled a lot of this information for you, so it is worth checking there first. Local councils also keep this data. In recent years a number of people have set up small businesses that specialize in formatting census data into computer software packages that your centre can purchase. Some health departments have also developed these software packages. These are particularly useful if you want a map which indicates, for example, the spatial distribution of an ethnic group in your area. Another group which is very active in this field is population geographers. Population geography departments at tertiary institutions may provide you some service or consultation in this area.

　　When you wish to focus on the data directly pertaining to the population's health you may need to search a range of sources. Mortality (cause of death by age, sex and place of residence) data are collected by the ABS. Hospitals supply health departments with morbidity data (based on diagnosis and length of stay). Natality statistics (births, birthweights and deaths before one year of age) are collected by the National Perinatal Statistics Unit. Again, your regional or state office of the health department may have collated these data for your area.

To get a more comprehensive view of the whole population's health (and not just illness episodes serious enough to cause admission to hospital) the ABS also undertakes population health surveys on an occasional basis. Data collected include current medical conditions, frequency of visits to medical practitioners, current medications, and days lost off work due to illness and disability. The ABS also has conducted a number of specific-purpose surveys to determine, for example, the levels of childhood immunization and also the extent of disability in the population. The National Heart Foundation (NHF) has undertaken population surveys of coronary heart disease risk factors. The Australian Institute of Health (AIH) in Canberra is responsible for collating and analysing health data to monitor progress towards Australia's national health goals. The Institute also keeps track of the research undertaken by some of these major organizations.

Table 3 summarizes some of the main data sources for different types of data.

After you have consulted all the existing data on your community, some of the issues first raised by other people with you in Step 1 might be put into perspective. For example, contrary to popular view, prosecutions for illegal drug use in the area may be among the lowest in the state. Adolescent pregnancy rates may be among the highest. However, no new light may be shed on some problems, such as social isolation of the elderly, The established data sources may also yield new issues. For example asthma admissions may be higher than state average. You may need to clarify some of these issues further before you attempt to determine health priorities from among them.

Usually the choice lies between attempting to gather community opinion about health problems more systematically and, alternatively, focusing on a single target group or issue and collecting more data to elucidate the situation. With the example we have given above you may decide to survey the elderly and their caregivers. Alternatively, you could decide to cast about more widely for views on community needs from a larger sample of residents and service providers.

At this point you must not forget that your region or area may have developed a policy on the sort of data that must be gathered in needs assessment. In the USA, for example, the PATCH programme (Planned Approach to Community Health) routinely collects morbidity and mortality data, risk factor prevalence data from a random household telephone survey and community opinion leader data from a survey of key informants for each community committed to this particular process of health promotion planning. [4] Data from all three sources contribute to the decision about what the health priorities should be. A number of Australian examples of comprehensive approaches to needs assessment and programme planning have also been reported in recent years. [5,6]

Table 3. *Types of information and where to get it.*

Type of Data	Examples	Source of Data
Demographic data	age sex family size country of birth	ABS
Social indicator data	education levels income occupation employment status marital status	ABS
Health status mortality	cause of death by age, sex, place of residence	ABS AIH
morbidity	admissions to hospital (diagnosis and length of stay)	state health department
natality	births, birth weights, deaths in first year of life	National Perinatal Statistics Unit, AIH
other	illness episodes, medications, doctor consultations	Australian Health Survey, ABS
	risk factor prevalence	National Heart Foundation
	child abuse	community services department
	domestic violence	local crime statistics
	cancer incidence	state cancer council

Activity
Assume that you have decided to collect data from a sample of community residents about their opinion of community health needs. How would you go about this?

Feedback
Self-completed questionnaires or interviews with individuals or groups of people at one time ('focus groups') could be conducted. Your sample could be randomly selected households or alternatively you may decide to consult those people in the community who may be well placed to advise you on community needs such as health workers, child care

workers, pharmacists, youth workers, leaders of community organizations and so on ('key informants'). Later chapters in this book cover techniques in questionnaire and survey design and how to run a focus group.

How much data should you collect? Bearing in mind that your primary responsibility is programme delivery and not research, at this stage we recommend that you collect no more data than you could possibly analyse by yourself using a pocket calculator. Community risk factor surveys of the type mentioned earlier need large sample sizes to get accurate results, usually more than 200 to 300 people. This is a major undertaking requiring substantial resources (statistical backup, computing, etc.). If you feel that your initial enquiries justify this sort of investigation your energies might be better spent putting together a submission for the additional resources and expertise to do this rather than attempting to undertake something like this on your own.

Step 3 Presentation of the findings

Everyone who has contributed information and advice to your project so far should be invited to view your progress. You should also be thinking of the groups, individuals and organizations who may play a key role in the direction and success of subsequent intervention planning. The community has a right to participate in the process that has been initiated and their participation is likely to determine whether the programmes that eventuate are culturally relevant and have the community's interest. Even if the work so far has been directed by a community group rather than a single health worker, there is a need at this point to open up the process for wider scrutiny.

The participation process will be significantly enhanced if the data are presented clearly and in a fashion likely to generate comments and analysis. Compare, for example, two sets of identical data on causes of death in Western Sydney. If you presented the data as they appear in Table 4 at a public meeting, chances are that the only comments you would get would be from other health workers in the audience who have had some training in data analysis and interpretation. In this case you could have had your discussion back at the office. On the other hand, the same data presented as in Figure 1 are easy to understand and invite comments and discussion from a wider audience.

You should attempt to make your presentation as attractive and stimulating as you can to promote interest and discussion of your findings. Perhaps you could show some slides of your interviewing and some of the agencies and people you spoke to to make your data appear more real. Consider putting your key points into a friendly looking pamphlet. Have on hand a full report for presentations at more formal meetings. An excellent example of how to present survey findings to the community is contained in the report of a survey conducted

Table 4. *Leading causes of death in the Western Metropolitan Health Region of Sydney, 1979–1982.*

Cause of Death	Number of Deaths		Standard Mortality Ratio	
	Males	*Females*	*Males*	*Females*
acute myocardial infarction	4028	2562	115.85	110.47
malignant neoplasms				
lung	1130	274	113.52	111.87
colon	420	404	99.94	97.83
breast		499		98.06
stomach	218	145	117.72	118.95
cerebrovascular disease	1290	1896	93.30	94.61
other heart disease	556	669	91.31	90.74
motor vehicle accidents	876	290	104.08	98.61
bronchitis, emphysema and asthma	311	159	98.40	103.03
suicide and self-inflicted injury	306	115	84.69	92.44
pneumonia	188	175	105.16	108.44
diabetes	184	217	115.56	125.99
chronic liver disease	244	94	88.79	84.75
other respiratory diseases	681	261	124.14	114.16

source: ABS

by the Southern Vales Community Services Research Unit in Noarlunga, South Australia.[5]

Step 4 Determining priorities
Now for the hard bit! Unfortunately there never seem to be sufficient resources to design interventions for all the needs you have identified. Decisions have to be made about which ones should be tackled first. Who makes these decisions? Is it you and your colleagues in the health department? Or are you working for a more broadly based community health planning group? How will you reach a decision? These are the issues you must sort out now.

Activity
Let's say that the findings of your work so far have thrown up several issues. These are high rates of adolescent pregnancy in your community, high cost of medical care, inadequate public transport and a high level of smoking. What criteria would you encourage people to think

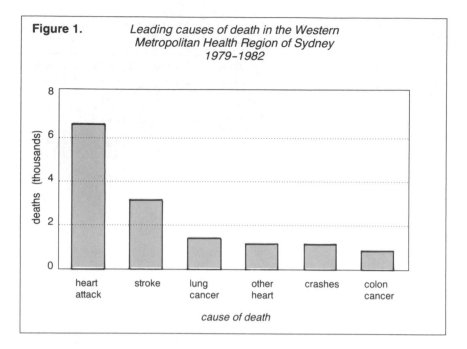

Figure 1.   Leading causes of death in the Western
Metropolitan Health Region of Sydney
1979–1982

about when you invite them to consider which health need should
have top priority?

Feedback
There are a number of points you might consider.[7]

Prevalence—
   Is the problem widely experienced?

Severity—
   Is the problem debilitating or does it only cause minor inconven-
   ience? What does it mean in terms of potential years of life lost,
   quality of life and health care costs?
Selectivity—
   Does it affect one group of the population in particular, say a
   group that is chronically disadvantaged and least able to cope
   without assistance.
Amenabilty to intervention—
   Is it known that interventions have succeeded with this problem?

   To make these kinds of decisions you will need to draw on your
experience and reading of what sorts of interventions are known to
work with the different problems you may be considering. For example, we know that lung cancer is caused by smoking which is a

problem amenable to intervention, but that Alzheimer's disease is not as yet considered preventable. This will affect your choice of problem. You may need to take some 'time out' to review the literature and seek advice. Ultimately you will also need to consider, in a more general sense, if the benefits of your intervention with a particular health problem will outweigh or justify its costs. In choosing priorities people's own values, opinions and experience will come into play as well. Only frank and open discussion will bring these under scrutiny.

To help a group of people reach a decision about the priority health problem or need you may decide to talk it out or you could choose to employ techniques which will facilitate the reaching of a general consensus. Rules for consensus decision making have been put together and tested by Hall.[8] You could also try a method called nominal group technique where people in a group rank different problems and follow a structured process whereby most are eliminated until discussion tends towards agreement.[9] Voting can be conducted but this tends to highlight differences and generally the result is that the people who hold the minority view become disgruntled and less involved in the subsequent proceedings. This is a reminder that the time and care you put into this part of the process will yield later benefits in terms of continued participation and enthusiasm. The work you do in facilitating the identification of a priority health need requires patience and skill and illustrates that needs assessment is not simply research.[3]

Again, it should be noted that if this step is frustrating you because the community is not picking the problems that concern you most then the issue lies with you choosing the wrong starting point in the needs assessment process. If you truly can work or develop programmes only in a particular field (such as cardiovascular risk reduction or cancer education) then your starting point in needs assessment is in the next stage, which starts with the health problem as given. Steps 1 to 4 in needs assessment are best conducted by health workers who can truly place themselves in a position to respond to local community needs. This is not to say that cardiovascular disease and cancer are not important health problems, only that when stacked up against other local community issues a democratic process cannot guarantee that they will be selected first. These are issues which will be discussed again later in the chapter.

At the end of Stage 1 you should have a statement about the top priority health problem, its magnitude and the group experiencing the problem. For example, 'teenage pregnancy rates 4 times that of the national average' or '50% of girls aged 13 to 16 are smokers'. It is important to state the magnitude of the problem from the beginning as this starts you thinking about the goal you might set in relation to reduction of the problem. Also, without acknowledging the size of the problem in the first instance you will not be able to measure the degree of your success in overcoming it.

Stage II   Analysis of the Health Problem

Armed now with a health problem and a target group you are set on your way towards planning your intervention. Before you can start that, however, you need to understand more about what is going on with this particular health problem and you need to collect some more information! It is always tempting at this stage to charge in and start developing programmes because of the amount of time you have already put in so far without seeming to have much to show for it. Do take some time and care with this second stage of the process though, as it is designed to help you avoid many of the mistakes that were made in the early days of health promotion when poorly conceived programmes failed.

The focus of the second stage of needs assessment is on developing a close and detailed analysis of who is experiencing the problem and why. A detailed profile of the target group is put together to help you later direct your intervention precisely to where it is most needed. The analysis draws on the experience of your target group and the people associated with them as well as the published reports of similar programmes or of people investigating similar problems with similar groups.

Step 5   Literature review

Let's assume that the problem that has been chosen is teenage pregnancy. Published papers should be searched for (1) reports on factors known to be contributing to the problem and (2) types of interventions that have already been tried and tested, and their success rates. This gives you a view of where the field stands and how your own intervention might contribute. A later chapter in this book outlines specific techniques you should employ in effectively and efficiently accessing the literature. You also might consult any databases that have been put together to list and sort programmes in this area, such as the national computer database on health promotion programmes HEAPS (which is coordinated through state health departments).

Step 6   Describe the target group

If it has not already been specified, you must now describe the target group for your intervention in more detail. This should include demographic characteristics such as age, sex, ethnic composition and also such factors as place of residence and education level achieved. It is important to be able to list these as later in your process evaluation you will assess the characteristics of the group that was actually reached by your programme and determine how well they represent the intended target group. Another reason for specifying this group in detail is so that health workers in other areas can compare your group with their own population before they decide to duplicate aspects of your intervention. Finally, the nature of the target group will also influence the style of your intervention.

By the end of Stage I in needs assessment you may already have quite a lot of detail on your target group, depending on the source of data used to identify this health priority. However, if this is not the case, further investigation will be required. For example, if the problem of adolescent pregnancy has been chosen you may need to do a small survey of medical record data to collect the details you need. This might include, for example, the age groups, ethnic background, location of residence and so on.

Step 7   Explore the health problem

Activity
Let's say that you will be designing a programme to reduce the adolescent pregnancy rate in your area. You know from the literature that other people have found the following to be important factors that seem to be contributing to the problem: poor contraceptive knowledge, low self-esteem and few alternative cultural role models. Before you set out to design an intervention for your own group what would you need to determine? What sort of information would you want to collect and how would you go about doing so?

Feedback
Research evidence can help to guide your thinking about a problem, but nothing beats talking to your own target group and the people associated with them. This is because the contributing factors or the emphasis in your group may be different. The literature may guide your line of questioning, but at this stage it would be wise to leave your questions fairly open and be led by the direction in which the group takes you. This may uncover some unexpected beliefs and associations. In Western Sydney, for example, health educators have reported that unless they had undertaken this step in the planning of a community nutrition programme for Australian women of Anglo origin they never would have discovered that many of their group considered rice to be an 'ethnic' food.[10]

An ideal method for exploring the sorts of factors that seem to be associated with contributing to the health problem is the focus group. This is the name for a group interview, where the leader leads the group through a fairly loose series of open-ended questions and invites discussion and comment. The leader should encourage expression of a range of views and create the sort of climate in which people feel safe to reveal their thoughts and feelings. A later chapter in this book is devoted to how to run a focus group with adolescent pregnancy as an example focus.

Table 5. *Framework for assessing the factors associated with or contributing to the health problem or health behaviour.*

Factor	Some Examples
Individual	• attitudes • knowledge • values • beliefs • self-esteem • self-efficacy • health locus of control • literacy
Social	• role models • social support • social desirability • cultural norms
Environmental	• physical environment • pollution • housing • transport routes • water supply
Health service	• availability • accessibility • sensitivity/ acceptability to target group
Financial	• cost of services or preventive care • financial incentives for prevention
Political	• political self-efficacy • opportunites for participation in decision making • policies on health and equity
Legislative	• safety regulations • environmental protection laws • regulations regarding exposure to hazardous materials • school immunization laws

The sort of data you collect in this step will significantly determine the focus and style of your subsequent intervention, which is the subject of the next chapter. Table 5 may help prompt you to cast about widely for the sorts of factors that may account for your health problem.

Step 8   Analysis of factors contributing to the health problem: causal pathways

By now, as a result of your investigations, you should be able to list all the sorts of things that might be contributing to the health problem or issue of concern. If we stay with the adolescent pregnancy example, these might be:

- poor use of contraceptives
- limited knowledge about contraceptives
- barriers to purchase of contraceptives (shyness at the chemist)
- cost of contraceptives
- low self-esteem
- lack of sense of belonging or a satisfying social role ('I need a baby to give me something to look after and something to do')
- financial support as a single mother ('at least I'm not a dole bludger')

- using contraceptives is seen as negative ('it's not romantic, guys think that you must have sex a lot if you are on the pill')

What we have to do now is sort these factors into a logical order that will help tease out the causal pathways leading to the problem of adolescent pregancy, that is, the series of factors and events that seem to lead up to the problem. We will also introduce some terms which will be used again in the chapter on programme planning.

First of all we identify those things which will be called **risk markers**. These are factors which signal where the problem is occurring. They identify the target group. These factors are associated with the occurence of the health problem, but do not necessarily directly contribute to it.

Risk markers for adolescent pregnancy:	girls aged 14–17 years; low socioeconomic group; Anglo-Australian origin

The next category to put into order is the risk factors. These directly account for why the problem is occurring.

Risk factor for adolescent pregnancy:	having sex without contraception

The third category is the contributing risk factors. It might help to think of these as being 'further down the line' or lower down in the causal pathway. These factors contribute to or account for the risk factor (in this case sex without contraception).

Contributing factors to the risk factor: (here, contributing to sex without contraception)	poor knowledge; cost of contraceptives; barriers to purchase; attitudes to contraception; attraction of becoming a mother; financial support to supporting mothers

The next task is to sort these factors into three classes. The first class is the factors which predispose a person to behaving in a certain way or predispose a situation to occurring. These are called **predisposing factors**. They include things such as knowledge, attitudes and beliefs. The second class of factors are **enabling factors**. These are factors which enable a behaviour or a situation to occur. For example, knowledge of the association between lung cancer and smoking may predispose a person to quit smoking, but the availablity of smoking cessation programmes enables a person to practise skills and techniques in quitting. The final class of factors are **reinforcing factors**. These are factors which reward or punish the carrying out of a behaviour or the maintenance of a situation. For example, in relation to smoking, a reinforcing factor would be the reduction in insurance premiums for non-smokers.

Why bother sorting contributing factors into predisposing, enabling and reinforcing? Because later on in your programme planning you will see that unless your intervention is focusing on factors in all three classes it is very unlikely that you will bring about and maintain any change in a situation. In other words, 'you have to cover all your bases' for the programme to work. So what may seem a tiresome process will be well worth the effort.

Some readers may recognize at this point that we have slightly modified the definition of predisposers, enablers and reinforcers as originally put forward by Lawrence Green and his colleagues.[11] A comparison of this adaptation of Green's approach to the original model is discussed in Appendix 1.

Back to adolescent pregnancy. If we now classify the factors contributing to the risk factor (of having sex without contraception) into the three classes predisposing, enabling and reinforcing, you will find that our example now looks like this:

RISK FACTOR: *having sex without contraception*

CONTRIBUTING RISK FACTORS

1. Predisposing
- *attitudes to contraception*
- *knowledge about contraception*

2. Enabling
- *high cost of contraception*
- *barriers to purchase of contraceptives at the point of sale*

3. Reinforcing
- *value/belief that it is OK to get pregnant—it gives you a role in life*
- *financial support to single mothers seen as better than the 'dole'*

What may happen now as you look back over your work is that you start to see the character of what a comprehensive intervention in this area would be. You should also start to realize the sorts of changes in all three areas that would have to occur if the strategy is to work. For example, adolescents can be made aware of the importance of contraception but still not feel comfortable about buying contraceptives.

Sometimes it is difficult to distinguish between predisposers, enablers and reinforcers and you may find that other people classify factors differently. It is a matter of judgement. The important thing is to start thinking about how the factors interrelate and what combination

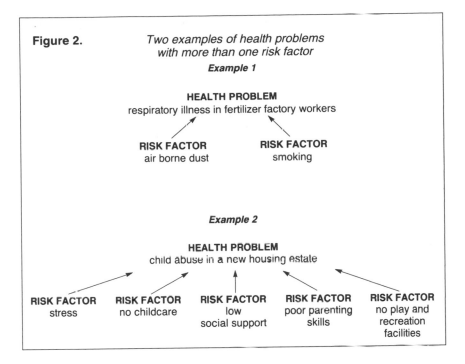

Figure 2.   *Two examples of health problems*
with more than one risk factor
Example 1

HEALTH PROBLEM
respiratory illness in fertilizer factory workers

RISK FACTOR   **RISK FACTOR**
air borne dust   smoking

Example 2

HEALTH PROBLEM
child abuse in a new housing estate

RISK FACTOR **RISK FACTOR** **RISK FACTOR** **RISK FACTOR** **RISK FACTOR**
stress   no childcare   low   poor parenting   no play and
                                      social support   skills   recreation
                                                                          facilities

of changes in the contributing risk factors would have to be made to bring about a change in the risk factor. It is always simpler to think about the relationships as being linear (one leads directly to another), but this is not likely to be the case.

Before we go on you should note that in the adolescent pregnancy example that we have chosen, there was just one major risk factor (having sex without contraception) and it describes a health behaviour. What about when there is more than one risk factor for a health problem? Consider the examples in Figure 2.

Below each risk factor in each example we could begin to add contributing factors and sort these into the predisposing, enabling and reinforcing factors. As you will see in the next chapter a single programme can be developed to address several risk factors at once. So, in relation to Example 2 above, a community development programme to foster social support networks, provide play opportunites and lobby for more facilities could be undertaken. However, in relation to the first example you could see that a simple stop smoking programme run for fertilizer factory workers may be insufficient. If health workers in a community centre offered this sort of programme they would need to be confident that their efforts were being complemented by the work of others to tackle the on-site problem of airborne dust.

At the end of this step (its length does signify its importance!) you should have a clear idea of the sort or factors you are going to attempt to target in your intervention. Exactly how you do this is discussed in the next chapter. The final thing you need to do, however, is see how the community and other agencies and organizations are presently situated in relation to the area that has been chosen.

Step 9   Reassess and strengthen community resources

Many communities we work with have already developed the structure and machinery to address their health needs. In setting yourself up to plan a new intervention you should first be aware of existing resources and programmes. Many health interventions should be planned in partnership with the community.

We are also reminded by Goepinger and Baglioni that too often the focus of needs assessments is on community deficits rather than community strengths.[12] In other words, instead of focusing simply on needs, you should make a careful assessment of community strengths and capacities. You should take the opportunity to assess the existing skills, knowledge, expertise, history in getting things done and so on and build on this. You may also take this opportunity to enlist the support and involvement of different organizations and members of your target group for the planning of your intervention if they are not already part of the process. With this type of emphasis, Step 9 is really part of Step 1.

Check Point

By the end of needs assessment you should have:

- a health problem of agreed high priority
- an indication of the magnitude of the health problem
- a target group with a set of clearly identifiable characteristics (risk markers)
- a set of risk factors and a set of contributing risk factors sorted into predisposers, enablers and reinforcers
- an indication of community resources to be involved in the health planning process
- commitment from a range of groups and parties to bring about change.

Issues in the Assessment of Community Need

Community Involvement

Community involvement in health promotion planning is widely supported. Australia's Better Health Commission adopted the view that communities are entitled to be involved in decisions affecting their health and health services.[13] However, in health promotion, community involvement appears to have different meaning and emphasis depending on your overall philosophy and approach. For example, in some community development approaches, the planning process is directed almost entirely by the community and the process is intended to foster equity and fulfilment of community goals. Community development is a method of empowerment and the nature of the health promotion programmes that may be developed is possibly less important than the process itself. On the other hand, with some other approaches to health promotion planning and development, involvement of the community appears only to be a device to smooth the way for programme implementation and improve the likelihood of programme success.

This book does not attempt to cover models, philosophies and theories of health promotion. We wish to remind you, however, of the need to reflect upon and clarify your own approach as this directly affects the style of your needs assessment and the emphasis you will give to different steps and components. It affects your notion of successful needs assessment. It also affects your notion of success in programme evaluation.

Conflict

When you start talking to many different groups, people and organizations you will soon find disagreement and conflict among them. Sure, you can avoid this by staying back in the office, but back there groups of health professionals may also disagree about what needs should be addressed first.

There is no easy way to deal with this. Some of the techniques for conflict resolution and consensus decision making skills mentioned earlier in this chapter may be of assistance. As a general rule things will be a lot easier if you first encourage people to articulate why they feel a certain way and what criteria they are using as the basis of their decision, rather than letting them all argue over what they have already decided. Get people to reveal the interests behind their position, as this may make different positions easier to reconcile. It is important that people's values and experience are out in the open. You should encourage each person to make a contribution and acknowledge this even if the final decision does not go 'their way'.

You should also be very clear about when a decision is going to be made as a result of a democratic process in contrast to when a decision is going to be made by a health worker, planner or policy maker in the light of the views expressed by others. It is important not to confuse the two. We are not advocating one method over the other here. Your style of approach is your responsibility, depending on your agency and your overall approach to health promotion. We simply wish to point out the importance of understanding which is which.

Inadequate Data

Sadly, you may find that when you set out to gain a comprehensive picture of the community's health you are prevented from doing so because of inadequate data sets. It is easier to get access to some data than to other data. You may find, for example, that you can fairly easily find out what the cause of death is for people in your community but data such as minor illness episodes or self-perception of health are collected much less regularly. This is a serious problem if perceptions of community need tend to become bound by inadequate sources of data. That is, when we perceive as problems only those things which we can readily measure, then the health promotion programmes we develop reflect this limitation.

Fortunately, the situation is changing and it will continue to do so if more and more people make demands on the organizations responsible for national health surveillance. In particular we need routine assessments of factors pertaining to the measurement of health in the more general and positive sense rather than simply mechanisms to record major illness events.

Ethical Responsibilities

When you ask a health worker why they might hesitate to do a needs assessment, you may get an answer such as: 'In case the community asks for something I can't do anything about!' This is a real possibility in needs assessment. There are many examples where health workers have found that the services usually provided by their centre (relaxation, weight control, stress management, nutrition advice, etc.) only come up on the community's list of priorities as fifth or twelfth after issues such as traffic noise, street lighting or pollution. This is a humbling experience!

Before you set out on a needs assessment you must anticipate what can be done in response to the priority health needs that might arise. Health workers funded in specific areas, such as cardiovascular risk reduction or drug abuse, may find themselves in a clear dilemma should a community decide not to choose these health problems first. Unless you are really in a situation to help a community respond directly to the needs you have helped them to identify, it is unethical to conduct a needs assessment under this guise.

There are two useful approaches to this problem. Firstly, intersectoral planning in health promotion is being practised more widely. This means that at the outset health workers are formally linked in networks and planning groups with health surveyors, local government engineers, local industry and so on. This means that the capacity to respond to a diversity of issues is considerably increased. The World Health Organization initiative, 'Healthy Cities' in Australia will give us an opportunity to observe and learn from this approach.[14]

Secondly, it has been widely observed that after you respond to the community's more urgent and pressing needs, they may come round to considering those issues that may be of utmost concern to health professionals. Meredith Minkler, for example, has described how a community development worker for a family planning agency first had to assist the community to deal with issues concerning garbage collection and drug pushers in school playgrounds before she had the credibility to gain the community's interest and support to deal with family planning issues.[15] The experience of the PATCH programme in the USA has been similar. Only after concentrating on issues of local community concern did the community turn its attention to those issues that coincide with national interests, such as heart disease, cancer and motor vehicle accidents.[4]

References

1. Denton LR. Noc Noc—What's there? Three basic considerations in evaluating community mental health centre programs. *Canada's Mental Health* 1976,24 (2):19–23.

2. Bradshaw J. The concept of social need. *New Society* 1972; March: 640–643.

3. Weinstein MS, Evans D. A community's health education needs must be defined. *Health Education* 1983;Fall:2–7.

4. Kreuter M. CDC's Planned approach to community health (PATCH). *Proceedings of the 12th world conference on health education*. Available from Health Education Bureau, 34 Upper Mount Street, Dublin 2, Ireland 1987;2:710–714.

5. Southern Vales Community Health Service Research Unit. *Noarlunga's Health. Apathy or Action*. A report to the community of a survey. S.A. August 1985.

6. Queensland Department of Health. Epidemiology and Prevention Unit. *Dalby Health 2000. A community based approach to disease prevention and health promotion*. Qld Department of Health, October 1988.

7. Wilson D, Wakefield M. *Priorities for Health Promotion in South Australia*. Working Paper No. 1. Health Promotion Branch, South Australian Health Commission, 1986.

8. Hall J. Decisions. Decisions. Decisions. *Psychology Today* 1971;November: 51–54, 86–88.

9. Delbecq AL, Van der Ven AH. A group process model for problem identification and programme planning. *Journal of Applied Behavioural Science* 1971;7(4):466–492.

10. Degling D. Unpublished paper presented at the Heart Health Symposium, Gosford, March 1990.

11. Green LW, Kreuter MW, Deeds SG, Partridge KB. *Health Education Planning. A Diagnostic Approach*. Palo Alto, California: Mayfield Publishing Co., 1980.

12. Goepinger J, Baglioni AJ. Community competence: a positive approach to needs assessment. *American Journal of Community Psychology* 1985;13:507–523.

13. Better Health Commission. *Looking Forward to Better Health Vol 1*. Canberra: Australia Government Publishing Service, 1987.

14. Baum F, Brown V. *Healthy Cities Australia: From Vision to Reality*. Sydney: Australian Community Health Association, 1987.

15. Minkler M. Ethical issues in community organization. *Health Education Monographs* 1978;6(2):198–210.

Further Reading

Bell RA, Sundel M, Aponte JF, Murrell SA, Lin E. *Assessing Health and Human Service Needs. Concepts, Methods, Applications.* New York: Human Science Press, 1983.

Davis DD. Participation in community intervention design. *American Journal of Community Psychology* 1982;10(4):429–445.

Lareau LS, Heumann LF. Inadequacy of needs assessment of the elderly. *The Gerontologist* 1982;22(3):324–330.

Warheit GJ, Bell RA, Schwab JJ. *Needs Assessment Approaches: Concepts and Methods.* Rockville, Maryland:US Department of Health, Education and Welfare, National Institutes of Mental Health, 1971.

Wutchiett R, Egan D, Kohaut S, Markman HJ, Pargamant KI. Assessing the need for needs assessment. *Journal of Community Psychology* 1984;12:53–56.

Chapter 3
PLANNING YOUR PROGRAMME

OBJECTIVES

By the end of this chapter you should be able to:

1. Define the goal, objectives and sub-objectives of your programme.
2. Explain how the goals, objectives and sub-objectives are derived from your analysis of the health problem.
3. Explain how goals, objectives and sub-objectives are tied to evaluation.
4. Demonstrate how to select a strategy and define a strategy objective.
5. List the steps in programme planning.
6. Develop and pre-test programme components.

How do we make a health promotion programme take shape? What strategies should the programme use? What should the programme set out to achieve?

Rational programme planning involves working through these questions and more. The purpose of programme planning is to devise a programme that is appropriate to the health problem and the identified target group, within the resources available, and which will have the best chance of bringing about the desired change. Programme planning also provides an opportunity to stop and rethink some of the usual assumptions we carry with us about the sort of action we think is required. The final plan should be precise enough for a person other than you to pick it up and implement it.

This last point is very important. The detail which we suggest in your programme plan is necessary to avoid the possibility that different staff members in your health team interpret and implement the plan differently. You need to be sure that deviation from the plan is for a good reason (such as a change in the target group's needs) and not simply because people in your centre or agency misunderstood exactly what was required. A detailed programme plan also lets you thoroughly work through the logic of your programme, to draw on accepted theory and experience about what is likely to work. Finally, a detailed programme plan documents the programme fully so that should your evaluation show that the programme is effective, people in other centres can duplicate your programme and bring about wider benefits.

Building up a Plan

Goals, Objectives, Sub-objectives and Strategy Objectives
Let's look at why it is important to distinguish between words which many of us usually do not stop to think much about.

Activity
Consider the following case study:

> A community nutritionist is designing a programme which uses drama as a way of educating preschool children about healthy foods. The 'objectives' for the programme are listed below
> 1. To show young children the sorts of foods which are the most healthy to eat
> 2. To make learning about health fun

What is wrong with the way these 'objectives' for the programme are stated?

Feedback
This is a common way of setting out what the programme aims to do, but the problem with the way these 'objectives' are stated is that they describe what the health worker does in the programme and not what changes he or she hopes to bring about in the target group.

For example, the programme may show young children the sorts of foods which are the most healthy to eat (so the 'objectives' may be deemed as achieved) but this may make no difference to children's subsequent knowledge or awareness of which foods are healthy and which are not and what they subsequently eat. In other words, objectives must be stated in a way that identifies the changes which you want to see as the result of the programme, and not simply describe what you set out to provide or deliver or conduct. Unless objectives are stated in this way you may be fooled into saying that your objectives have been achieved, and your programme is successful simply because you ran the programme and not because it worked.

In fact, the 'objectives' described in the example above are what we term *strategy objectives*. Strategy objectives describe what you do in the programme, that is, what the programme provides as opposed to what the programme achieves, which are the real objectives. *Objectives* describe what changes you want to bring about in the target group (here preschool-aged children). An objective for the programme in the example might be:

> To increase by 30% the proportion of kindergarten children who eat a healthy balanced diet

The figure of 30% is part of a requirement to be specific about the objective which we will come to again later.

The *goal* of the programme is what you want ultimately to achieve by running the programme, in this case, say, a reduction in the proportion of primary school children who are obese. Again note how the goal, like the objective, describes a change in the target group. As you will see later, the goal also has to be stated very specifically.

It follows that achievement of the objectives should lead to achievement of the goal. In other words, the objectives and the goal illustrate a causal pathway, with the goal being the change in the health problem or condition that motivated you to design an intervention. A programme may have more than one objective. What about the sub-objective? A *sub-objective* is what has to happen before an objective can be achieved. It is further down the pathway from the objective. For example, if your objective is about a change in behaviour, your sub-objective might be about a change in a factor which you feel is a prerequisite for the change in behaviour. So, in the example we have given so far, a sub-objective may be about the proportion of children who can distinguish healthy foods from overly fatty foods. That is, it could be about nutrition knowledge.

However, in many programmes you don't have sub-objectives. This is because the objective may not be something which has prerequisite parts. This often happens when you state the goal of the programme to be a change in behaviour (like eating or smoking) and the objective to be a change in knowledge or attitude. It then becomes difficult to take the issue further into a sub-objective. However, when the goal is a change in health status, you often find that you can plan a programme down to the level of sub-objectives or even further.

How the Goals, Objectives, Sub-objectives and Strategy Objectives Relate to your Evaluation

What you state as your goal, objective, sub-objective and strategy objective relates directly to what you measure in your evaluation, which is why goals, objectives and strategy objectives must be carefully worded.

Because objectives (and sub-objectives) and goals concern the changes you want to see in your target group, whether or not these changes occur are the focus of your evaluation of programme effects. Impact evaluation focuses on the initial impact of the programme. That is, did the programme achieve its objective (and sub-objective)? Outcome evaluation focuses on subsequent or longer-term effects. That is, did the programme achieve its goal? Process evaluation focuses on the activity of the programme and how well the programme was delivered. This corresponds to the strategy objectives.

HOW PROGRAM COMPONENTS RELATE TO EVALUATION

PROGRAMME GOAL	*is measured in*	Outcome evaluation
PROGRAMME OBJECTIVE (AND SUB-OBJECTIVE)	*is measured in*	Impact evaluation
STRATEGY OBJECTIVE	*is measured in*	Process evaluation

So, in relation to the preschool nutrition example discussed previously, the outcome evaluation would be about reductions in obesity in primary school children. The impact evaluation would measure a change in diet. The process evaluation would measure how well you were able to conduct your programme: did the children like it, was it fun, was the material presented clearly, did they understand it and so on.

How Goals, Objectives and Sub-objectives relate to your Analysis of the Health Problem

Remember in the second stage of needs assessment when the analysis of the health problem broke it down into risk factors and contributing risk factors, which were then subdivided into predisposers, enablers and reinforcers? This is to help you set your objectives and sub-objectives.

RELATIONSHIP OF GOAL, OBJECTIVE AND SUB-OBJECTIVE TO ANALYSIS OF THE HEALTH PROBLEM

GOAL	*corresponds to*	Health problem
OBJECTIVE	*corresponds to*	Risk factor
SUB-OBJECTIVE	*corresponds to*	Contributing risk factor

Let's see how this works in relation to a real health problem.

EXAMPLE 1

HEALTH PROBLEM	Excessive exposure of school children to ultraviolet light	GOAL	To reduce exposure of school children to ultraviolet light
RISK FACTOR	Children don't wear hats	OBJECTIVE	To increase the proportion of children who wear hats
CONTRIBUTING RISK FACTORS	Children don't like wearing hats (predisposing)	SUB-OBJECTIVE	To increase the proportion of children who like wearing hats
	Hats are not supplied by the school (enabling)		To make hats free for school children
	Hats are not a compulsory part of uniform (reinforcing)		To make wearing of hats compulsory for school children

Let's see how the objectives and sub-objectives are altered when you pick a different risk factor for the same health problem.

EXAMPLE 2

HEALTH PROBLEM	Excessive exposure of school children to ultraviolet light	GOAL	To reduce exposure of school children to ultra violet light
RISK FACTOR	Not enough shade in school playgrounds	OBJECTIVE	To increase the amount of shade in school playgrounds
CONTRIBUTING RISK FACTOR	Parents and teachers not sufficiently aware of risk of sun exposure (predisposing)	SUB-OBJECTIVE	To increase the teachers' and parents' knowledge of risk of sun exposure

Insufficient funds to build shelters (enabling)	To acquire $10 000 for shade shelters
Education Department has no policy on shade areas (reinforcing)	To have shade protection incorporated into Education Department school policy

You might like to think of other risk factors for the same health problem.

From examples 1 and 2 you can see just how carefully you must consider your approach to a health problem to make sure that you will design a programme which will encompass sufficient factors and be likely to work. You can see from this example that the usual first impulse 'Wearing Hats is Fun' campaign on its own would be a waste of time. This is why analysis of the health problem and thoughtful planning is worthwhile. It tells you what complementary activities would have to occur (either directed by yourself or others) to bring about a change in the health problem.

Specifying your Goals, Objectives and Sub-objectives

It is not sufficient to simply state in your goal 'To reduce head injuries from bicycle accidents' because we are left wondering exactly what programme success means. A 20% reduction over 10 years? A 10% reduction over 3 years? A reduction in injuries in children? In all age groups? In all regions or areas? Goals, objectives and sub-objectives must be specified by time, person, place and amount. But how do you know how much change to aim for? How do you know what time period to select?

The basic answer to these questions is that you set your goals and objectives from your understanding of the nature of the health problem and the target group. The following points outline how you apply your understanding to setting and expressing goals, objectives and sub-objectives.

Place
Place is easy to identify. This refers to the geographical location, organization or setting in which the programme is to take place.

Person
This usually refers to the target group. If you're not planning for change in individuals or groups of people, but for legislative, environmental or organizational change, specify which organization or which

aspect of the environment instead of which person or group of people. Give details—specify the age group, the sex, the interest group, etc. of the people who are your target group. Be equally as specific with organizational, legislative or environmental goals—name the type of organization, the level of government and so on.

Time

Time refers to the point by which you expect to see the desired change and is usually expressed as a period after the beginning of the programme (e.g. within 6 months of the beginning of the programme); or as a period after the end of the programme (e.g. within one year after the end of the programme), or by the end of the programme, depending on the sort of programme and the effects you are looking for. It could also be in terms of milestones, such as 'by the year 2000', which has become a popular approach.

Amount

This is expressed as either:

1. increasing or decreasing the proportion of people carrying out the behaviour or practice of interest, e.g. to increase the proportion of men aged 35 to 60 in Lazytown who exercise three times a week, by 30% within a year of the beginning of the programme; or
2. increasing or decreasing the average frequency of a behaviour or factor of interest, e.g. to increase the average number of times per week that men aged 35 to 60 in Lazytown exercise, from 1.5 to 3 times per week within one year of the beginning of the programme.

This illustrates an important point. It may make a difference clinically whether your focus is on the average number of times a population carries out a behaviour or on the proportion of people in the population who carry out the behaviour in the desired fashion.

For example, in relation to smoking we know that the impact on lung cancer and cardiovascular disease will only occur if we increase the proportion of non-smokers in the community and not simply reduce the average number of cigarettes smoked in the community (which may or may not correspond to an actual change in the proportion of non-smokers). A goal stated in the latter manner may be easily achieved and measured, but it may have minimal clinical importance. That is, it may have no effect on reducing the incidence of illness. Consult an epidemiologist or biostatistician if you need extra help.

Some guidelines on how much change by when

1. There are often national goals and targets set by the government, e.g. a national reduction in dietary fat of 5% across the population by the year 2000.

2. Look at what amounts and timeframes other people have achieved. Check the literature for other programmes like yours (including pilot programmes). Use a similar timeframe and aim to do as well as or better than these, but again make sure that your target group has similar characteristics to the people in the other programmes.

3. Ask funding bodies, colleagues and people whom you may wish to make referrals to your programme, what degree of change or success they consider to be important or significant.

4. Don't forget to check any work on the same health problem or other health problems that has been done with your target group, to assess their readiness to be involved and their amenability to change. Talk with as many people as your can—colleagues, community leaders and members of the target group.

5. Compare the size of the health problem in your community with surrounding communities or the average for your area, state or the country. For example, if you have 30% more pregnant teenagers in your community than the national average, it would be unrealistic to have as your goal a reduction in teenage pregnancies to below the national average. While this might be a desirable outcome, you are not likely to achieve a reduction of this magnitude with one programme.

6. Check for natural fluctuations in the size of the problem. Say for example that the number of hospital admissions for asthma varies by about 5% from year to year. You would need to find a reduction greater than this to be sure that your asthma medication education programme worked and any reductions you found were not caused by chance, so you would set your goal accordingly. Some fluctuations are contingent on changes in the environment, such as season, geography or other factors. Motor vehicle accidents always increase during holiday periods. If you don't take these factors into account when setting how much and by when, you won't know whether your programme caused the reduction in accidents or whether there were fewer accidents because there were no holidays at that time.

7. If you are going to run a programme such as 'Living with diabetes' that competes with another established programme you will need to show that yours is more successful to persuade people to support it.

8. Don't forget to check what you wrote down as risk markers and characteristics of your target group. Do you think these will have a particular influence on the success the programme? For example, if your national target for increasing exercise is 30% and you are working with a disadvantaged community where there are few facilities for exercise, you might not want to aim as high as the national target.

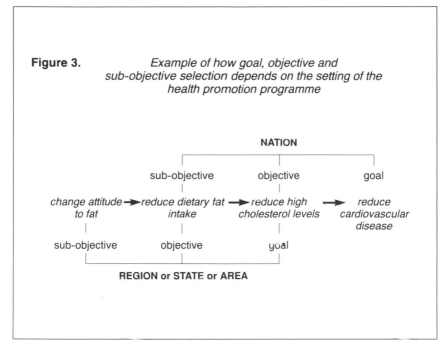

Figure 3.   *Example of how goal, objective and sub-objective selection depends on the setting of the health promotion programme*

Of course, sometimes you may not find any stated guidelines and there may not be anyone to help you either. If you are working at the community level you can take all of the above information into account and set the goal yourself. What you often end up doing is taking a 'best bet' approach—there's always a first time.

What Goals and Objectives will be the Focus of your Programme?

You can see that once you choose a particular health problem, say lung cancer, heart disease or substance abuse, there are a range of behaviours, conditions or factors that you can set out to change. The ones you choose are determined by your agency or setting, your location, your access to resources (time, staff, skills, equipment, venues, etc.) and what you are likely to be able to do well. You may be in a position to set as your goal a change in health status. Your programme would then set out to improve health status and your evaluation would be set up to measure this. Alternatively, you may only be able to set your goal as a change in behaviour, say in smoking or dietary intake, or a change in environmental hazards, such as water purity or safe road crossings and this is what you would measure in your evaluation.

Depending on where people work and their access to resources, one person's goal may be another person's objective, as indicated in Figure 3. For example, at a state or regional level, health workers may be setting up programmes to reduce high cholesterol levels in the community. At a national level, health workers may be monitoring how this affects the national incidence of heart disease.

A Note on Target Group and Intervention Group

During most programmes in health promotion you will work with the people experiencing the health problem (target group). However, in some situations, in order to bring about the desired change in the target group you will need to work with another group whose behaviour or attitudes affect the target group.

EXAMPLE

To reduce the number of accidents involving young children and electrical outlets you may need to educate the parents as to the importance of installing safety power points. You would measure achievement of your goal (outcome evaluation) as a reduction in the number of deaths from electrical accidents among the children (the target group). You measure achievement of your objective (impact evaluation) as change in parents' knowledge and attitude toward safety (intervention group).

Selecting Strategies and Activities

At the Curtin University of Technology in West Australia, the materials in the Distance Learning Programme in Health Promotion contain the statement:

> The three most common words in discussing the relevance of health promotion strategies are ' . . . it all depends'[1]

What then follows is a useful discussion of how different methods work best in different settings. For example, lecture and discussion formats and group-based education suit school-based settings. Worksite environments may use group techniques plus analysis of and changes to the environment itself. Institutional settings (such as hospitals) can use group methods and organizational development. Local action programmes can use community development and organization. Large-scale community programmes may also include a media focus.[1]

Inevitably, your setting and your philosophy in health promotion affects the sort of strategy you will choose. It may have already influenced how you analysed the health problem, what you consider as contributing factors and so on and therefore what you have set as your goal and objective. In Chapter 1 we pointed out how some health promotion programmes have a focus on individual self-management for health, while others have an emphasis on collective action for community health. So too do programmes differ in analysis of the health problem and in the approach to solutions.

You need to be conscious of your preference and orientation as you will be unlikely to see a need for rational planning if your actions are virtually predetermined. The planning process should provide an opportunity to see new solutions to problems and appreciate new perspectives.

If you want to use a strategy that you are not familiar with, you will need more information than is provided here to make sure that your strategy is theoretically sound. You may decide to draw on the skills of other people and resources to help you decide. For more information about strategies in health promotion consult the reading list at the end of this chapter.

Strategy Objectives and Strategy Activities

Strategy objectives state what your programme is going to provide and deliver, whereas your sub-objectives or objectives describe what you hope your programme will achieve (and your goal describes what you hope will result from this achievement). So strategy objectives are about running education programmes, conducting media campaigns, organizing collective action at a community level and so on.

A single strategy objective can bring about the achievement of multiple objectives or sub-objectives as shown in Figure 4.

Strategy activities are what you actually do to meet your strategy objective. They are the component parts of your strategy objective. So the strategy activities in an assertiveness training programme may be role plays, discussions, relaxation exercises and so on. Figure 5 illustrates the relationship between sub-objectives (or objectives, if your programme plan has not been reduced to sub-objectives), strategy objectives and strategy activities. Figure 6 shows a worked example for two different strategy objectives to promote exercise in a community.

Development and Pre-testing of Programme Materials

Programme materials are the aids and accessories you need to implement your programme. They may include handouts, leaflets, equipment such as a sphygmomanometer and audiovisual materials such as videos or films. Materials must be pre-tested or tried out with the target group to make sure that they will be acceptable and suited to their needs. This is particularly important if you have 'imported' materials or 'packages' from a programme outside your own area and you are adapting it to your own group.

The next chapter on process evaluation has techniques for assessing the quality of programme materials and you should consult this sec-

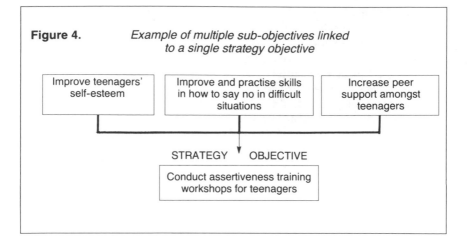

Figure 4. *Example of multiple sub-objectives linked to a single strategy objective*

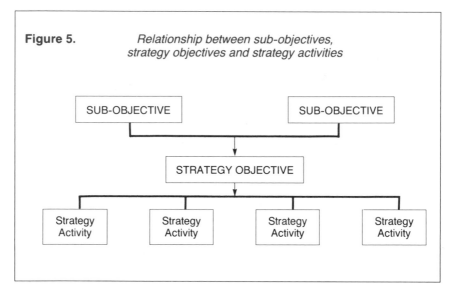

Figure 5. *Relationship between sub-objectives, strategy objectives and strategy activities*

tion. If you are using group leaders for your programme you should conduct a trial run or session or at least take the opportunity to observe how they work with another group.

Training of Staff

Your programme may be conducted by a range of different people: say, those who may screen participants and assess health risks, those who provide health counselling, people who lead groups or education sessions, even the receptionists in your centre who may have the first

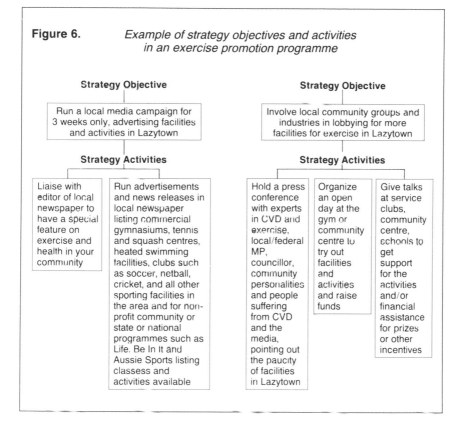

Figure 6.   *Example of strategy objectives and activities in an exercise promotion programme*

Strategy Objective

Run a local media campaign for 3 weeks only, advertising facilities and activities in Lazytown

Strategy Activities

Liaise with editor of local newspaper to have a special feature on exercise and health in your community	Run advertisements and news releases in local newspaper listing commercial gymnasiums, tennis and squash centres, heated swimming facilities, clubs such as soccer, netball, cricket, and all other sporting facilities in the area and for non-profit community or state or national programmes such as Life. Be In It and Aussie Sports listing classess and activities available

Strategy Objective

Involve local community groups and industries in lobbying for more facilities for exercise in Lazytown

Strategy Activities

Hold a press conference with experts in CVD and exercise, local/federal MP, councillor, community personalities and people suffering from CVD and the media, pointing out the paucity of facilities in Lazytown	Organize an open day at the gym or community centre to try out facilities and activities and raise funds	Give talks at service clubs, community centre, schools to get support for the activities and/or financial assistance for prizes or other incentives

contact with participants. All of these people need a good understanding of the programme and a thorough grasp of their role. Even if your coworkers are using a community development approach and there is no set programme format, you need to be sure that people are comfortable in their role, able to deal with situations that present themselves and able to signal when they feel not up to the task in hand.

Training sessions organized at the beginning of the programme should bring together programme staff to discuss programme rationale and procedures and to practise skills involved in the programme, such as role plays of health screening and so on. You need to make sure that people undertaking the same tasks do so uniformly, so that programme success as much as possible is attributed to the content and techniques of your programme and not just the peculiarities of any individuals associated with it.

After a period of intense training, which may take days or weeks, depending on the style of programme, training sessions should evolve into regular programme staff meetings, so that people can refresh their skills and raise new issues associated with running the programme.

Figure 7.   *Example of a checklist for organization of a meeting*

☐ Venue

☐ Date and time

☐ Resources—films/video/posters

☐ Speaker

☐ If using a speaker: confirmation in writing of date, time, venue and subject

☐ Advertising: circular to group members; posters or handouts at health centre, community aid, local shops, doctor's surgery; telephone or address for enquiries

☐ Audio-visual and other equipment: projector, slide/tape, butcher's paper, black/white board, overhead projector, carousel, screen

☐ Refreshments: facilities for boiling water, cups, coffee, tea, food

☐ Child care: room, toys, books, changing table, toilet, drinks, fruit, childminders, etc.

☐ Transport, parking, access for the disabled

☐ Person to handle enquiries and record bookings

☐ Person to introduce the film or speaker

☐ Handouts, if being used

☐ Thank-you letter to speaker or a small gift

This is particularly important to allow you to review and make changes to the programme as necessary and for maintaining staff morale.

Implementation and Administration

From the moment you commence training sessions you may need to develop a programme manual which lists procedures in the programme and decisions made subsequently about any modifications or changes in policy once the programme has started. Good documentation will prevent arguments later about how particular problems were resolved. Your manual will also help new staff who may join the programme later in its development.

Implementation of the programme will also involve advertising the programme and details associated with the budget and resources to keep the programme running. Figure 7, for example, outlines a checklist of tasks associated with running a single meeting.

For a very large programme, you may need an organizational chart of programme activities, when they occur and who is responsible for each of them.

Summary: The Steps in Programme Planning

The following list of steps in programme planning will give you an overview of the process we have described.

1. Assess your resources, consider your setting and agency and what you should be able to achieve.
2. Set goal.
3. Set objectives and (if necessary) set sub-objectives.
4. Select strategy (ies).
5. Set strategy objectives.
6. Devise strategy activities.
7. Develop and pre-test programme materials.
8. Train staff.
9. Set up administration, advertising and record keeping procedures.
10. Implement programme.

A Worked Example: The Plan of a Heart Health Programme

Figure 8. *Analysis of a health problem*

Health Problem

Elevated levels of serum cholesterol among blue-collar males aged between 45 and 64 years; average in excess of 5.5 mmol/L

Risk Factor Associated with Health Problem

High intake of dietary fat

Contributing Factors

Predisposers	Enablers	Reinforcers
• poor knowledge of what healthy foods are • no-one interested in cooking • poor understanding of meaning of the term cholesterol • no real interest in heart health	• unavailability of healthy take-away foods • cost and convenience primary determinants of what food is selected and consumed • high dependence on take-away foods as part of regular diet	• mixed health messages from media • doctors don't actively counsel patients about diet and heart disease • cultural norms about males and red meat

Figure 9.   *The plan of a heart health programme*

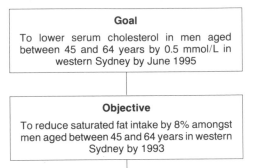

Goal

To lower serum cholesterol in men aged between 45 and 64 years by 0.5 mmol/L in western Sydney by June 1995

Objective

To reduce saturated fat intake by 8% amongst men aged between 45 and 64 years in western Sydney by 1993

Sub-Objectives

- increase knowledge of relationship between dietary fat and serum cholesterol and its importance in reducing cardiovascular disease by 50% by end of the programme
- increase the proportion of healthy food choices at take-away food outlets by 20% within 6 months of beginning of programme
- increase the proportion of low-fat meals served at home by 25% by the end of the programme
- increase knowledge of food content labels in order to facilitate healthier food selection by 50% by end of the programme
- increase proportion of people who like low-fat/low-cost food by 20% within 1 year of the programme

Strategy Objectives

- establish a heart disease and cholesterol risk factor screening, counselling, information and referral service for target group
- train staff in the screening procedure
- provide intensive dietary intervention programmes for those unable to modify own diet
- provide worksite education sessions on heart health for target group
- provide community-based programmes, heart health education programmes including a healthy fast-food choices programme and an education programme on food labelling
- provide low-fat/low-cost cooking programmes for the target group and/or their wives
- increase opportunities for tasting low-fat foods
- contact the managers of fast-food outlets and negotiate the provision of at least one healthy choice
- lobby food standards committee to simplify the labels on food
- train general practitioners in counselling and supporting patients in heart disease prevention

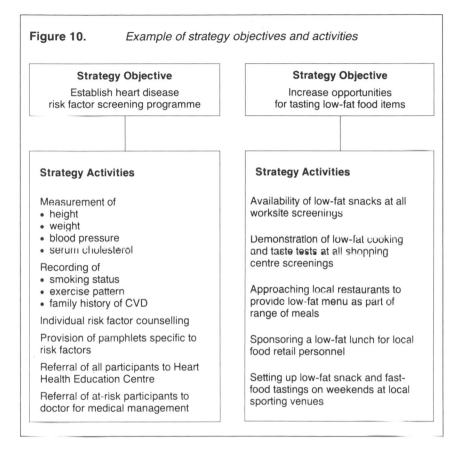

Figure 10.   *Example of strategy objectives and activities*

Strategy Objective

Establish heart disease
risk factor screening programme

Strategy Objective

Increase opportunities
for tasting low-fat food items

Strategy Activities

Measurement of
• height
• weight
• blood pressure
• serum cholesterol

Recording of
• smoking status
• exercise pattern
• family history of CVD

Individual risk factor counselling

Provision of pamphlets specific to
risk factors

Referral of all participants to Heart
Health Education Centre

Referral of at-risk participants to
doctor for medical management

Strategy Activities

Availability of low-fat snacks at all
worksite screenings

Demonstration of low-fat cooking
and taste tests at all shopping
centre screenings

Approaching local restaurants to
provide low-fat menu as part of
range of meals

Sponsoring a low-fat lunch for local
food retail personnel

Setting up low-fat snack and fast-
food tastings on weekends at local
sporting venues

A whole-community programme to improve heart health is an example of where you would need a careful plan to devise an appropriate intervention and to coordinate all the different activities involved. The following is an example of how a plan for such a programme could develop. In this example we will first assume that a needs assessment generated the analysis of the health problem shown in Figure 8.

Elevated levels of serum cholesterol is the health problem of interest. Figure 9 outlines the beginnings of your plan.

In the example in Figure 9, as you can see some of the strategies of choice are screening, counselling and education, referral, community education and social marketing.

Now see in Figure 10 how two of these strategies have been broken down even further into strategy activities.

Reference

1. Egger G, Spark R. *Health promotion strategies and methods* 583. Distance Learning Program. Graduate Diploma in Health Promotion. Department of Health Promotion. School of Community Health. Curtin University of Technology. West Australia. 1989;99.

Further Reading

Bonaguro JA, Miaoulis G. Marketing: A tool for health education planning. *Health Education* 1983;14(1):6–11.

Dignan MB, Carr PA *Program Planning for Health Education and Health Promotion.* Philadelphia: Lea and Febiger, 1987.

Green LW, Anderson CL. *Community Health.* St Louis: Times Mirror/Mosby, 1986.

Green LW, Kreuter MW, Deeds SG, Partridge KB. *Health Education Planning. A Diagnostic Approach.* Palo Alto, California: Mayfield, 1980.

Green LW, Lewis FM. *Measurement and Evaluation in Health Education and Health Promotion.* Palo Alto, California: Mayfield, 1986.

Ross HS, Mico PR. *Theory and Practice of Health Education.* Palo Alto, California: Mayfield, 1980.

Rossi RJ, McLaughlin DH. Establishing evaluation objectives. *Evaluation Quarterly* 1979;3(3):331–346.

Chapter 4
WHAT TO MEASURE FIRST: PROCESS EVALUATION

OBJECTIVES

By the end of this chapter you should be able to:

1. Define the three types of evaluation—process, impact and outcome evaluation.
2. Identify the main questions addressed in process evaluation.
3. Assess how well your programme has reached your target group.
4. Assess what programme participants think of your programme.
5. Monitor the implementation of your programme, and determine whether all your programme activities have been carried out as planned.
6. Determine the quality and appropriateness of programme materials and other aspects of the programme (such as audiovisual materials and group leaders).

Your first obligation in process evaluation is to make sure that the programme you planned has really been set up and run the way you intended. This is not as crazy as it sounds. For all sorts of reasons, what you set out to do on paper may change. The sort of people who attend your programme may be different from the original group you had in mind. Your staff may vary the session format a little to fit in with new needs. Equipment or films may not be available or may change. People attending may not like what you do so you may make minor improvements or major alterations. You may even find that you simply can't carry out what you intended because in practice it's just too hard!

Process evaluation covers all aspects of the process of programme delivery and includes things like looking at session content, attendance and what people think of the programme. This sort of feedback usually gives specific information which will help you improve the programme and develop it into a better form. For this reason process evaluation has also been called 'formative evaluation'.

Unless a programme is getting to the right people, is being implemented the right way and people are satisfied with it, you would not expect the programme to work. That is why you must do process evaluation before you do any other sort of evaluation that assesses the programme's effects. It would be silly to go looking for effects when the programme itself is not functioning optimally.

Even when you are confident that the programme is in its best form and running the way it should, you can keep using the techniques of process evaluation just to keep a watch on the way things are going. This is referred to as quality assurance; making sure that the quality of programme delivery meets standards of good practice.

In this section we will illustrate the range of different techniques you can use in process evaluation. Once your programme is in a stable form, we will recommend what sort of techniques you should use routinely and what techniques you should use just occasionally to make sure that the quality of your programme is still meeting your initial expectations.

Types of Evaluation

Process evaluation:	measures the activities of the programme, programme quality and who it is reaching.
Impact evaluation:	measures the immediate effect of the programme (does it meet its objectives?).
Outcome evaluation:	measures the long-term effect of the programme (does it meet its goals?).

As you can see, process evaluation is just the first of three different types of evaluation that can be undertaken. Impact and outcome evaluation are dealt with in Chapter 6.

It is very important that these three forms of evaluation are done in sequence so as to avoid premature evaluation. Premature evaluation is evaluating something before it is likely to work. For example, it would be premature to rush in and look for long-term effects of a programme before you know that the programme is running the way it should, is reaching the right people and is having the expected initial effects. Unfortunately, many people make this mistake: they conclude falsely that because the desired changes were not observed the programme did not work. A more likely explanation is that the programme was not correctly implemented.[1] This would be detected in process evaluation. Doing process, impact and outcome evaluation in the correct sequence will help you avoid looking for higher order effects before you have observed initial ones.

The Main Questions in Process Evaluation

There are four main questions you should ask about your programme during process evaluation.

1. Is the programme reaching the target group? Are all parts of the programme reaching all parts of the target group?
2. Are participants satisfied with the programme?
3. Are all the activities of the programme being implemented?
4. Are all the materials and components of the programme of good quality?

Assessing Programme Reach

Activity

You have set up a programme to involve teachers and parents in teaching kindergarten children how to use a pedestrian crossing, after widespread publicity about the idea of the programme, it is now running in 5 kindergartens in your area. The goal of the programme is to reduce pedestrian accidents in the 4 and 5 year age group. How would you assess whether or not your programme is reaching the target group?

Feedback

First of all, you could use the attendance figures for participating kindergartens to tell you the number of children involved in the programme. Let's say the number is 110. To make more sense of this figure you need to know the total number of children in your area or municipality who are in your target group. Let's say that the Australian Bureau of Statistics' figures tell you that the size of this group is 2750. You can then deduce that you are getting to 4% of your target group, or 1 in 25. This will allow you to decide, for example, that in the second year of the programme you would like to aim to get to 1 in 15 children and you might change the advertising and resourcing accordingly.

It is also possible to determine programme reach for media-based health promotion programme. Media campaigns are common tools in health promotion programmes, with health messages appearing on radio and television spots, in mobile caravans/displays and in the

Table 6. *Proportion of people who had encountered and correctly interpreted an immunization message in a South Australian immunization campaign.* *

Immunization message	Proportion of people
Tetanus	41.3%
Rubella	25.2%
Measles	25.2%

* Data published by Macdonald and Roder.[2] Reproduced with permission.

widespread distribution of pamphlets and posters. To assess the public awareness of an immunization education campaign in South Australia in 1981, health workers surveyed 409 adult shoppers at a major shopping centre. Seventy-seven people (18.8%) said that they recalled the campaign without any prompting from the interviewer. Subsequently, the names of a range of different campaigns were read out to the people surveyed and following this 40.8% could recall a specific advertisement about immunization. Table 6 gives further detail about how different messages about immunization were recognized. This information gives campaign planners valuable insight into the nature of their messages, which may allow them to make improvements.

Of course, many health education and health promotion programmes have a number of components. For example, people may attend a cholesterol screening service in a shopping centre and those with high levels might be referred to a dietary and lifestyle programme run at the community health centre. The programme may be run across 4 sessions. After this people may be given a home dietary maintenance programme and then later come along to a follow-up session. You would not expect the programme to have its full impact unless enough people had been exposed to a sufficient amount of the programme.

A hypothetical example of the level of implementation of this programme is given in Figure 11. You can see that the health educator who collects this information and constructs this histogram at the end of the first time the programme has run would most certainly want to look at ways to reduce the programme drop-out rate. This would be addressed before he or she went on to look at overall programme effects.

Assessing Participant Satisfaction

Unless you have a very unusual programme you would expect people to have to like it, or at least value it, before you would expect it to have the desired effects.

Activity

You have been running a lifestyle programme which involves people attending 4 weekly sessions on nutrition, exercise and relaxation given

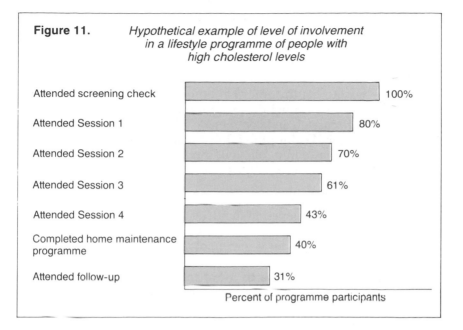

Figure 11. *Hypothetical example of level of involvement in a lifestyle programme of people with high cholesterol levels*

Attended screening check — 100%
Attended Session 1 — 80%
Attended Session 2 — 70%
Attended Session 3 — 61%
Attended Session 4 — 43%
Completed home maintenance programme — 40%
Attended follow-up — 31%

Percent of programme participants

at the local district hospital. How would you assess participants' satisfaction with the programme?

Feedback

There are a number of ways to do this. Let's look first at what to measure and then we'll talk about how to do it. There are 3 main types of things you can ask participants about.

1. Interpersonal issues. Do they feel comfortable in the programme? Do they feel that they are listened to and understood? Are the other participants friendly? Are staff interested, approachable, sincere?
2. Service issues. Is the programme venue convenient and comfortable? Is it easy to get to? Is the programme run at a convenient time? Are the facilities adequate? Is the programme too costly?
3. Content issues. Are the topics covered relevant? Interesting? Presented in the best way? Is the pace too slow or too fast? Is it too complex/easy? Are some things being left out or not covered in sufficient depth? Remember, you are not ready yet to assess whether learning has taken place. At this stage you just want to make sure that you are covering the right topics.

You can measure these things in a variety of ways, depending on what you think your group could cope with best. The most detail and privacy for participants is gained by distributing individual questionnaires for participants to complete. This is a good way to get anonymous feedback. However, this technique only works well with a group which takes to pen and paper tasks, and is obviously not good for people with reading or language problems. You need to allocate time for the task to be done (preferably in the group) and make sure that you get all the questionnaires back.

Another way to get this information quickly is to conduct a group interview, with you leading the group through your questions and recording their discussion and comments. 'Focus groups' are being used more commonly in health promotion and provided you do not think that airing their views in public will inhibit people, this is an efficient way to get feedback, especially as people can also comment on each other's views.

A tried-and-true group method of evaluating a programme (or even just a session) has developed in the drug and alcohol health education field in NSW. The group leader puts onto the wall a large sheet of butcher's paper and divides it into 4 columns. In the left hand column he/she writes down 5 or 6 items which are aspects about the programme that the group wants to comment on. These should be agreed on before proceeding. Commonly, the list would include the venue and facilities, the content of the speakers' presentations, the group leaders' skills, the group exercise or activity segments and maybe an 'other' category for comments of a general nature. The next column is headed up 'positive comments' or 'good things'. The third column is headed up 'negative comments' or 'bad things' and the last column is titled 'recommendations' or 'suggestions'.

The reason for this framework comes from the experience that people are much more likely to feel comfortable about giving negative feedback if they are given the chance to turn this criticism into a recommendation or something constructive.

To preserve anonymity the health educator or group leader can opt to allow 5 to 10 minutes for each person to complete the task individually. The leader then puts people into groups of 5 to 7 and allows 10 to 15 minutes for groups to pool their answers onto a group sheet. The group should be instructed that they should not try to reach consensus. What one person sees as a good point may be seen as a weakness by somebody else. That doesn't matter at this stage. The purpose is to record the information for later discussion. Finally, a spokesperson for each small group should present the group's comments to the larger group and to the group leader. If it is not too time consuming the health educator or group leader should write this onto the master sheet but, as the information has already been recorded, the real purpose of this is for discussion and to demonstrate that the leader has understood the remarks.

It is a good idea for leaders also to have positive and negative comments and make public any of their own suggestions. Again this demonstrates objectivity and encourages people to be less shy with their

Table 7. *Hypothetical example of evaluation of a half-day nutrition workshop, conducted within a menopause education programme.*

Component of Session	Positive Comments	Negative Comments	Recommendations
1. Content	• Interesting • Made relevant to daily routines • Not too 'medical' • Recipes and meal planning suggestions excellent	• Didn't cover role of vitamin and mineral supplements	• Have a section on main myths of menopause nutrition
2. Teaching	• Friendly • Not like a schoolteacher • Easy to follow	• Went too fast at times • Spoke too softly	• Slow down • Speak up
3. Film and leaflets	• Woman in film was believable • Leaflet gave information on where to get more advice and help	• Didn't like doctor in film	
4. Group discussion	• Lots of opportunity to ask questions	• Group too large for all to be involved	• Need to limit group size to 10
5. Venue—facilities	• Good access for public transport • Comfortable seats • Air conditioning	• Personal arrangements for child care difficult	• Need child-minding to be available
6. Other		• Not enough on weight control	• More on kilojoule content and weight loss advice

views. The whole exercise needs to be contained within a reasonable time (say 30 minutes maximum for longer sessions) so that it does not get too tedious. The leader should collect the pooled comments from each small group and use these as the basis of documentation. A hypothetical worked example of this method of assessing participant satisfaction is given in Table 7.

Figure 12.   *Medication education*
                    session recording sheet

Topic	Tally (one mark = 1 min)	Time spent in minutes	Proportion of total session time
1. Brand names and generic names of drugs and drug strengths	ⅢⅠ ⅢⅠ II	12	20%
2. Importance of directions	ⅢⅠ I	6	10%

Assessing Implementation of Programme Activities

It is one thing to count whether all your participants show up at all the programme activities. It is another thing to check your side of things and see whether you are actually running all the activities the way you said you would! To get started write down all the components (sessions, activities) of your programme and think about ways to record and count whether everything happens the way it should. For example, during a year of running preparation for parenthood programmes, did the people from the Child Safety Unit come and give a demonstration to each group on the use of baby capsules in cars? All sorts of last-minute problems may reveal that only three-quarters of the groups had this component. You would need to fix this before you start investigating the effectiveness of your programme on baby car restraint use. This sounds simple enough but in practice few people make the effort to have this information close at hand. So first of all just count up your activities to see whether enough things happened the way they should.

Another important thing to measure is the content of the educational group sessions that you might have in your programme. When you plan a session which is aimed, say, at improving the compliance of elderly patients with a range of medications they may be taking, you need to have a way of making sure that everything the pharmacist or doctor talks about is covered with the appropriate emphasis each time.

The process evaluation of a patient medication education programme at Lidcombe Hospital in Sydney involved the design of a method to record session content. An observer attended each session run by the pharmacist and recorded the amount of time spent on each of the topic areas. The format of the form designed for this is illustrated in Figure 12.

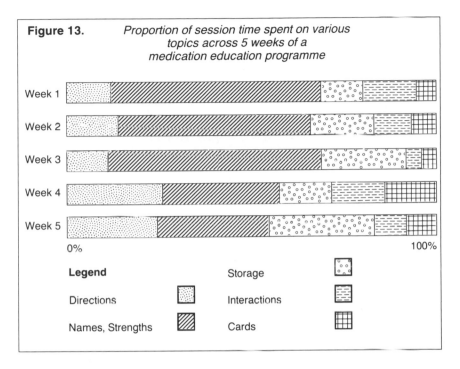

Figure 13. *Proportion of session time spent on various topics across 5 weeks of a medication education programme*

After recording this sort of information over a number of weeks it is possible to get a picture of the relative stability of the session and whether or not the appropriate emphasis is being given to each topic, relative to the overall goal or intention of the programme. Figure 13 is a series of bar charts which demonstrate the proportion of session time spent on 5 topic areas in the medication education programme across a period of 5 weeks.

At the end of Week 3, the programme designers got together and decided that less time should be spent on discussion of the names and strengths of drugs and more time on directions for taking medication. This is because the main compliance problem with the elderly is under-dosage rather than overdosage. The section on names and strengths is mainly directed at overdosage because people might double up unwittingly, not knowing that manufacturers are giving different names to the same drug. On the other hand, the section on directions covers things like taking drugs with meals to reduce the possibility of side effects, a common reason for underdosage. Weeks 4 and 5 in Figure 13 reflect the desired change in emphasis. This is a good example of how careful process evaluation leads to improvements in programme design.

668

EVALUATING HEALTH PROMOTION

STANDARD QUESTIONS FOR USE IN PRETESTING OF
HEALTH MESSAGES.[3*]

1. COMPREHENSION
   a) What was the main idea this (message) was trying to get across to you?
   b) What does this (message) ask you to do?
   c) What action, if any, is the (message) recommending that people take?
   d) In your opinion, was there anything in the (message) that was confusing?
   e) Which of these phrases best describes the (message)?
      — Easy to understand
      —Hard to understand

2. LIKES/DISLIKES
   a) In your opinion, was there anything in particular that was worth remembering about the (message)?
   b) What, if anything, did you particularly like about the (message)?
   c) Was there anything in the (message) that you particularly disliked or that bothered you? If yes, what?

3. BELIEVABILITY
   a) In your opinion, was there anything in the (message) that was hard to believe? If yes, what?
   b) Which of these words or phrases best describes how you feel about the (message)?
      —Believable
      —Not believable

4. PERSONAL RELEVANCE/INTEREST
   a) In your opinion, what type of person was this (message) talking to? Was it talking to:
      —someone like me
      —someone else, not me
      Was it talking to:
      —All people
      —All people, but especially (the target audience)
      —Only (the target audience)
   b) Which of these words or phrases best describes how you feel about the (message)?
      i) —interesting
         —not interesting
      ii) —informative
          —not informative
   c) Did you learn anything new about (health subject) from this (message)? If yes, what?

5. ARTWORK
   a) Just looking at the drawing (or picture), what do you think it says?
   b) Is there anything in this drawing (or picture) that would bother or offend people you know?

6. OTHER

Listed on this sheet of paper are several pairs of words or phrases with numbers 1 to 5 between them. I'd like you to indicate which number best describes how you feel about the (message). The higher the number, the more you think the phrase on the right describes it. The lower the number the more you think the phrase on the left describes it. You could also pick any number in between. Now lets go through each set of words. Please tell me which number best describes your reaction to the (message).

Practical	1	2	3	4	5	not practical
Too short	1	2	3	4	5	too long
Discouraging	1	2	3	4	5	encouraging
Comforting	1	2	3	4	5	harming
Well done	1	2	3	4	5	poorly done
Not informative	1	2	3	4	5	informative

*Reproduced with permission.

Assessing Performance of Programme Materials and Components

Chances are that in the work you do to assess participants' views and opinions of the programme, as described in the preceding sections, you will get comments on your materials—your leaflets, group leaders' skills and the like. There are also ways to assess these aspects more systematically.

Leaflets and Audiovisual Materials

Activity

In the development of a women's health programme you design and print a leaflet on breast cancer and the importance of breast self-examination. You want to develop a checklist of things you would ask about the leaflet to find out whether or not the leaflet is any good. The questions would be directed at the women who would read your leaflet. Remember that at this stage you are looking at the quality and presentation of the leaflet. You are not assessing learning as yet.

Feedback

A standard protocol has been developed for assessing the presentation style of leaflets and audiovisual materials before they are printed for distribution in final form. The US National Cancer Institute has designed a questionnaire (see box). You may like to use this questionnaire with your target group, or you may prefer to design your own, using the elements of the US instrument as shown below.

ATTRACTION:	Does the leaflet create interest? Catch people's attention? What do people like most and least about it?
COMPREHENSION:	Is the leaflet easy to understand? Is there anything confusing in the leaflet?
ACCEPTABILITY:	Is there anything offensive or irritating in the leaflet? Does it conflict with cultural norms (especially if translated insensitively into other languages)?
PERSONAL INVOLVEMENT:	Does the leaflet seem to be directed at the reader personally?
PERSUASION:	Is the leaflet convincing? Does it seem to persuade the reader to do something?

Readability

As well as pre-testing your target audience's reaction to your leaflet you can, to some extent, evaluate how easy it will be to comprehend. The SMOG Formula[3] is one way of estimating the difficulty of a piece of writing.

The formula is based on research which shows that—all other things being equal—texts with a lot of polysyllabic words require a higher reading comprehension level than texts with words of mostly one or two syllables. This makes common sense, of course, but it is easy to miss looking at the reading difficulty of a leaflet when deciding which one to use. If you use a health message that is hard to read, you might be preventing the very people you want to target from understanding your message.

The SMOG formula is simple and quick to apply. It yields an approximate reading grade needed to read and understand the text. This reading grade relates to average reading levels among the US population, so to help you interpret this for an Australian audience, we have SMOG-tested some well-known publications in Australia. The first two pages of the *Australian*, the *Sydney Morning Herald*, the *Daily Mirror* and *New Idea* were put to the SMOG test and scores for each appear in Table 8 and Figure 14.

This table can be used as a yardstick to help you work out what the SMOG score means and what SMOG level would be appropriate for your target group.

You can see that to get to a wide audience you would be well advised to pitch your health information at a SMOG score of 11 or 12 or lower.

Table 8. *Results of SMOG tests on four Australian publications.*

Newspaper or Magazine	Average number of Polysyllabic words for every 30 sentences.	(US Reading Grade required for comprehension)
Sydney Morning Herald	162	16
The Australian	137	15
The Daily Mirror	85	12
New Idea	63	11

Step-by-step SMOG formula

1. Mark off the text in three ten-sentence sections, one section at the beginning, one towards the end and one in the middle of the text. It doesn't matter if the sentences are long or short. If your text is only about thirty sentences long, or if it has less than thirty sentences, use the whole text as your sample.

2. Circle all the polysyllabic words (words with three or more syllables) in the thirty sentences you have marked off, including any repetitions of the same word. Add up the number of words you have circled.

3. If you have 30 sentences in your sample, go straight to step 4.
   If you have less than 30, find the average number of polysyllabic words per sentence by dividing the total number of words you circle by the total number of sentences. Then multiply your answer by 30 to get an estimated number of polysyllabic words per 30 sentences.

4. Find the nearest perfect square to the number of words you circled, and write down its square root.

5. Add a constant of 3 to the square root. The number you get is the SMOG grade, or the estimated reading grade level a reader needs to have reached in order to be able to read and understand this piece of writing.

Some further guidelines

- A polysyllabic word is one that has three or more syllables, e.g. elephant (3 syllables) elevator (4 syllables). Some words can be pronounced more than one way—e.g. sev-ral or sev-er-al. Choose the way you think is more common, or use a good Australian dictionary which shows pronunciation, such as the Macquarie Dictionary.

- Proper nouns should be counted too, if they have three or more syllables.

- Count hyphenated words as one word (e.g. mother-in-law or poverty-stricken). Sometimes the same words might be used but without hyphens (e.g. mother in law; poverty stricken). Don't worry about consistency or correctness, just take each instance at face value.

- Don't count headlines, sub-heads or quotes repeated from text.
- Abbreviations should be treated the way they are normally read aloud. In a sentence like, 'US Defence Force spokesman ...' the US is unlikely to be read out as 'United States', whereas the State of NSW is always read out as New South Wales. Do the same for acronyms, such as PATCH, WHO, etc. For example, in spoken language, the name UNICEF is used as one word, rather than the original title of United Nations International Children's Emergency Fund; whereas WHO is usually spoken of as the World Health Organization or 'Double-Yoo-Aitch-Owe'.
- Numbers should also be included in your calculations. Treat each number as one word, whether it is represented orthographically (e.g. forty-nine) or numerically (e.g. 49). Sound out the number to determine if it is polysyllabic.

Figure 14: (Opposite page) *A worked example of SMOG readability for 'Malice at the Palace'*

Step 1	Total no. sentences	30
Step 2	Total no. polysyllabic words	63
Step 3	(skip — there are 30 sentences in sample)	
Step 4	Nearest perfect square is 64, $\sqrt{64}$ =	8
Step 5	Add Constant	3
	Smog Score:	11

Group Leaders and Group Process

Health promotion programmes vary considerably in the type of role given to group leaders. In some programmes, such as fitness classes, the leader is an instructor or demonstrator. In other programmes—adolescents' personal development groups or self-help groups, say for bereavement—the group leader takes a much lower profile and tries to achieve the programme objective by facilitating a process of talk, thought and interpersonal support in group members. Obviously then, the way you set out to evaluate a group leader's performance will depend very much on the style and function of the leader's role.

When a group leader is functioning more directively, like an instructor, you can use questions like those developed by Miller and Lewis in 1982,[4] reproduced in the box. This questionnaire covers areas such as: the instuctor's friendliness, interest and ability to communicate and understand; the instructor's degree of organization and directiveness, whether he/she makes mistakes, moves too quickly, lacks attention to detail or accuracy; and the instructor's capacity to foster interpersonal support within the group.

MALICE at the PALACE*

The rivalry between Diana and Fergie has hotted up — even the number of children they'll bear has become an issue!

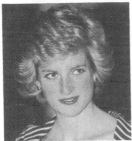

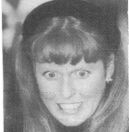

In public the Princess of Wales and the Duchess of York smile at each other and appear to be good friends.

But behind the scenes Fergie is determined to knock Diana off her pedestal as the most famous woman in the world.

"They don't squabble," says a palace insider. "But the rivalry between them is hotting up."

Not only is Fergie pulling out every stop in trying to prove that she is just as stylish and modern as her sister-in-law, but she wants to out do Diana by being a model mother too! By that, say insiders, she means that she is determined to raise a larger family than Diana traditionally the yardstick by which the royals judge their princesses.

Although Diana, 28, announced at the time of her wedding that she intended having at least five children, for the time being two seem to be sufficient.

Fergie, who turned 30 earlier this month, will catch up when her second child is born next March. In fact, it was with a sense of triumph that she called London journalists to announce her pregnancy.

Indeed, she was so eager to spread the news that the editors were given the information even before the Buckingham Palace press office!

Says Fergie to her closest friends: "I am determined to have a large family — six children at least!"

The ambition of the Duchess of York to be number one is being fought in every direction she can think of. For instance, when it came to what sort of home Prince Andrew and she should live in, the Queen offered Fergie a number of handsome properties. Some of these were among the best on offer in Britain. But to the astonishment of the royal family, Fergie turned down every one of them.

The palace source says: "The Duchess of York is not being greedy, but she just had to have a bigger home than her sister-in-law Diana. Finally, in despair, the Queen asked her daughter-in-law straight out, 'What exactly would you like as a home?' And without the slightest trace of embarrassment, she replied, 'I've set my heart on living in Frogmore'.

The Queen was astonished. This 17th-Century mansion is the greatest, most regal property in Britain outside Buckingham Palace. Members of the royal family are buried in its grounds. It was the home of the Duke of Windsor when he was Prince of Wales.

For Fergie it seemed a fair request. Her view is: "As Diana will become Queen one day, Andrew and I should be compensated by having a fine home."

Of course, this has not to come to pass, and Fergie has had to settle for the new home being built for her and Andrew at Sunninghill Park in Windsor. It may not be grand in the historic manner, but in opulence it looks like outdoing Diana's home Highgrove House in Gloucestershire — and it's just across the park from the Queen's residence at Windsor Castle.

One thing Fergie definitely knows she has got over Diana is personality.

Says one royal observer: "Fergie has the self-assurance and confidence to talk to people as though she is one of them. She has the common touch, thanks to her experience of life before she got married. Diana is far more shy and formal in her approach."

The Duchess is also much wiser in the ways of the world than Diana. She understands what reporters like to hear, whereas Diana is often tongue-tied in public and cannot think of the smart thing to say.

Thus, again and again, Fergie makes headlines. For instance, her words reverberated around the world when she joked after the birth of Beatrice: "Why my daughter is just like her dad — because she sleeps all through the night!" That comment made people everywhere smile broadly. It is something that Diana would never have dreamed of saying.

Fergie understands, too, how to win the affections of the royal family. She makes a point of riding with the Queen, knowing it's her favorite pastime, whereas Diana says she "hates horses".

❝Fergie has the common touch. Diana is far more shy and formal❞

One of the closest friends of the Duchess sums it all up with this: "I understand why Fergie's favorite song is that old American hit, Anything You Can Do, I Can Do Better."

Now, by becoming pregnant a second time, she is making it clear that she is catching up to Diana fast, and is determined to beat her every way she knows!

The only thing going against Fergie in her quest is that she's, for the most part, got to do it all on her own — basically because she thinks that only she knows best.

As one Palace courtier notes: "The only person she ever listens to is her father."

Each week they meet at Claridge's Hotel in London, and they chat almost every day on the telephone. Besides Major Ferguson and her husband (who is away most of the time, anyway), her other confidante is her former flatmate and now lady-in-waiting Carolyn Cotterell.

Even the views of old friends carry little weight. One says: "You try to say something to her, a few words of advice, you know, on a friend-to-friend basis, but she just knocks you back. She hates to be told what to do."

John Wood and Andrew Morton

NEW IDEA, 28/10/89 5

Assessments in this regard are carried out by group participants who rate the group leader's performance. An observer or member of staff could also sit in on a group and answer some of these items, but their presence may well change the dynamics of the group.

When the focus of a group is different, your approach to evaluating group leader performance should be different. When a group leader is involved in a programme where the emphasis is more on promoting interpersonal exchanges, you will probably want to include measurements of other sorts of dimensions. For example, the health worker may be attempting to set up a social support network for mothers of children who suffered cot death. The goal of the programme may be to prevent depression. Clearly it is not appropriate to assess the health worker's skill in terms of imparting educational information so much as it may be necessary to look at how well he or she performs as a group facilitator. In this sense, it is possible to measure the group environment (or 'group climate') created.

'Group environment' or 'group climate' simply refers to the feeling that is created in a group by the group members and the way they interact with each other. In the 1970s Rudolph Moos, a social psychologist, developed a series of scales to measure the social environment at work, in the family, in groups, in classrooms and in hospital wards.[5,6] The Group Environment Scale is a 90-item questionnaire that takes about 10 minutes to complete. Each item consists of a statement about the group and participants are asked to mark the item 'true' if the statement describes how they see the group or 'false' if the statement does not describe how they see the group. The dimensions measured by the Group Environment Scale and examples of items for each dimension are given in the box.

The Group Environment Scale and the other environment scales are psychological measures and as such can only be accessed in Australia via the test library of the Australian Psychological Society in Melbourne. If you are interested in these measures you first need to contact a psychologist or try the psychology department of one of the universities or tertiary institutions.

Clearly, not every group you conduct in a health education programme is going to set out to assist the participants in all of these subscales. It is possible to omit those items that are inappropriate to your context and thereby shorten the instrument considerably. Further, the cleverness of the instrument comes in when leaders use it to ask group members to complete the scale twice; once to describe how the group ideally should be and the next time to describe how the group really is. The group's overall degree of discrepancy between 'ideal' and 'real' is then used to change things to make the group environment more fitting. An illustration of this discrepancy in scoring is given in Figure 15. In this example the group has expressed a desire to be more cohesive with less leader control.

QUESTIONNAIRE FOR ASSESSING GROUP LEADER PERFORMANCE

Item	True	False
1. The instructor puts high priority on the needs of the class participants.	T	F
2. The instructor makes a lot of mistakes in class.	T	F
3. The instructor gives directions too quickly.	T	F
4. The instructor helps me feel that I am an important contributor to the group.	T	F
5. A person feels free to ask the instructor questions.	T	F
6. The instructor should be more friendly than he/she is.	T	F
7. I could hear what the instructor was saying.	T	F
8. The instructor is a person who can understand how I feel.	T	F
9. The instructor focuses on my physical condition but has no feeling for me as a person.	T	F
10. Everyone who wanted to contribute had an opportunity to do so.	T	F
11. There was too much information in some sessions and too little in others.	T	F
12. Just talking to the instructor makes me feel better.	T	F
13. The purposes for each session were made clear before, during and after the session.	T	F
14. Covering the content is more important to the instructor than the needs of the class.	T	F
15. The instructor asks a lot of questions, but once he/she gets the answers she/he doesn't seem to do anything about them.	T	F
16. The instructor held my interest.	T	F
17. The instructor should pay more attention to the students.	T	F
18. The instructor is often too disorganized.	T	F
19. It is always easy to understand what the instructor is talking about.	T	F
20. The instructor is able to help me work through my problems or questions.	T	F
21. The instructor is not precise in doing his/her work.	T	F
22. The instructor understands the content he/she presents in class.	T	F
23. I'm tired of the instructor talking down to me.	T	F
24. The instructor fosters a feeling of exchange and sharing between class participants.	T	F
25. The instructor is understanding in listening to a person's problems.	T	F
26. The instructor could speak more clearly.	T	F
27. The instructor takes a real interest in me.	T	F

Source: Miller and Lewis.[4]

SUBSCALE DIMENSIONS OF THE GROUP
ENVIRONMENT SCALE[5]

RELATIONSHIP DIMENSIONS

1. Cohesion

   The extent of members' involvement and participation in the group; of their affiliation and commitment to the group; of the help, manifest concern, and friendship displayed to each other. (Example: 'There is feeling of unity and cohesion in this group.')

2. Leader support

   The amount of help, manifest concern and friendship displayed by the leader to the members. (Example: 'The leader spends very little time encouraging members.')

3. Expressiveness

   The extent to which freedom of action and expression of feelings is encouraged. (Example: 'If ever members disagree with each other they usually say so.')

PERSONAL GROWTH DIMENSIONS

4. Independence

   The extent to which the group tolerates and/or encourages independent action and expression in its members. (Example: 'Individual talents are recognized and encouraged in this group.')

5. Task

   The degree of emphasis on practical, concrete, down-to-earth orientation tasks, decision-making or training. (Example: ' There is very little emphasis on practical tasks in this group.')

6. Self-discovery

   The extent to which the group tolerates and/or encourages members' revelation and discussion of personal detail. (Example: 'Personal problems are openly talked about.')

7. Anger and aggression

   The extent to which the group tolerates and/or encourages open aggression, expression of negative feelings and inter-member disagreement. (Example: 'Members are often critical of other members.')

SYSTEM MAINTENANCE AND SYSTEM CHANGE DIMENSIONS

8. Order and organization

   The degree to which the activities of the group are formalized, organized and structured; the degree of explicitness of group rules, norms and sanctions. (Example: 'The activities of the group are carefully planned.')

9. Leader control

   The extent to which the tasks of directing the group, making decisions, and enforcing rules are assigned to the leader. (Example: 'In a disagreement, the leader has the final say.')

10. Innovation

    The extent to which the group tolerates and/or facilitates diversity and change in its own functions and activities. (Example: 'The group does very different things at different times.')

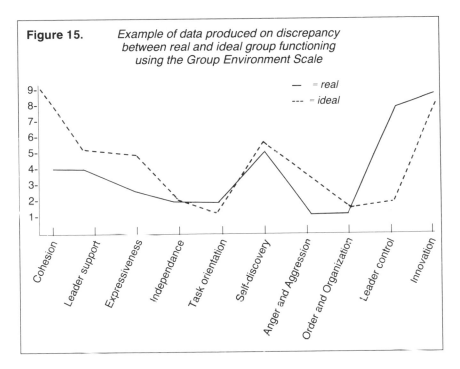

Figure 15. *Example of data produced on discrepancy between real and ideal group functioning using the Group Environment Scale*

Using this technique, the instrument itself does not dictate good or bad levels of functioning. This is defined by the participants themselves. The group then, on receipt of the feedback, tries to 'close the gaps'.

Of couse, not all groups will take to this level of assessment as it requires a degree of fascination with answering questions and gazing at graphs! You may choose to copy the elements of the dimensions and questions illustrated and simplify them into your own format.

How Much Process Evaluation should the Fieldworker do?

Each of the four main questions in process evaluation must be answered for each of your programmes. Your first responsibility when you set up a programme is to devise systems to assess programme reach, programme implementation and the quality of your programme materials and participant satisfaction. You then use the information to make changes to your programme. You evaluate these changes in a continuation of your process evaluation until you are satisfied at last that your programme is in an optimum and stable form. After this you can proceed to impact and outcome evaluation. Schematically this is illustrated in Figure 16.

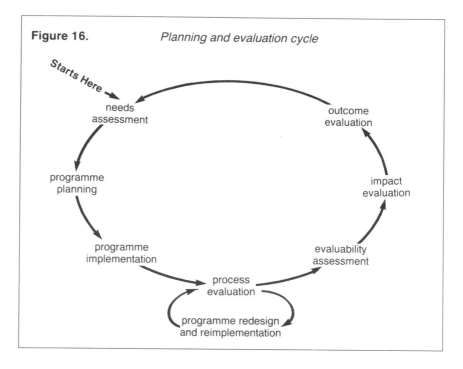

Figure 16. *Planning and evaluation cycle*

What happens after you reach that wonderful point when the programme is in its best form and you get the green light to move on to the evaluation of programme effects? Do you stop doing process evaluation? The answer is 'no', but the good side of it is that you don't have to do quite as much.

The reason why you still need to do some monitoring of the process of programme delivery is to make sure that the quality of your programme does not fall away. Some low-level, continuous and occasional monitoring will help you keep a check on things. It will tell you if you are still getting to the right target group, that your group leaders are still doing things well and so on. From a quality and standards viewpoint this information is essential. You also need to be sure of this when you move into impact and outcome evaluation.

As we will see later, impact and outcome evaluation measures the programme's achievement of objectives and goals—or short-term and long-term effects. This sort of evaluation is very involved. It is not done very often and it is usually costly. The results are important and usually remembered. You simply cannot afford to do an evaluation of this kind while running the risk that the programme reach or programme quality has dropped off. Although perhaps only a temporary problem, this can prevent you finding the programme effect you were after. Unfortunately, after showing that a programme has failed once (for whatever

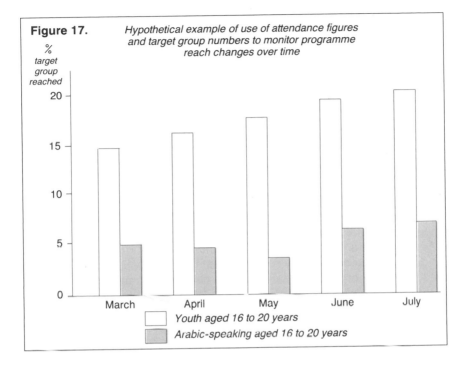

Figure 17. *Hypothetical example of use of attendance figures and target group numbers to monitor programme reach changes over time*

% target group reached

Youth aged 16 to 20 years
Arabic-speaking aged 16 to 20 years

reason), administrators are often reluctant to fund a second test of it. A potentially good programme may therefore never be fully appreciated or widely implemented.

Back to the question of how much process evaluation you should continue to do. From our experience, once you are satisfied with the programme's performance, as a matter of routine you should continue to collect your figures on attendance or programme reach, remembering to convert these into ratios whenever you have a reasonably good estimate of the size of your target group. To make the best use of this data you should devise a way of tracking your progress graphically, so that all the programme staff can see how well you are maintaining or improving the reach of a programme.

To graph programme reach data you should use a percentage scale because this will accurately display the increases you make (we hope) over time (see Figure 17). But reaching 4% of the target group may not sound as successful as reaching 1 in 25; and moving from 4% to 5% does not sound as much of a leap as moving from 1 in 25 to 1 in 20. So when you describe what's happening you might like to talk in ratios as well as percentages.

An example of the way you might do this is given in Figure 17. In this example a health and lifestyle education programme is being run at a youth drop-in centre. The target group for the programme is all adolescents aged 16 to 20 years, but the group of most concern is Arabic-speaking youth. You can see that by calculating monthly reach percentages for both of these groups the youth centre can track their progress across time and assess the impact of any new methods they devise to attract the adolescents to the centre. The procedure is helped if staff agree on a reach percentages for the year. If this percentage is not achieved special action is taken.

The other information that you must collect routinely is the proportion of programme components received by participants. A graph such as that produced in Figure 11 can also be adjusted to monitor progress across time in a series of graphs, as illustrated in Figures 18 and 19.

The data that we advise you collect routinely is in fact the sort of data about programmes that is often collected anyway. The difference is that we recommend you analyse, interpret and graph it, perhaps in a new way, to make the better use of it.

Some process evaluation we recommend you undertake just occasionally. This is because these sort of data are harder to collect in that they take up more time and effort. One class of data in this category is monitoring of session content. If you did this routinely it would drive you crazy! For this reason we suggest you do a random check on whether or not the appropriate material and emphasis is being given in sessions about once every six times a session is run (see Figures 12 and 13, pages 66 and 67). Evaluation of programme materials or components such as leaflets or group leaders is also very involved and we recommend that you do this once every 4 times the programme is run, but certainly not less than once a year.

It is important to remember that these recommendations for continued process monitoring apply to programmes that you have set up and have watched progress towards optimum functioning. What obligations do you have to process evaluation of programmes that you have imported from elsewhere? Unfortunately, you have to consider the fact that the glamour or success reported about the imported programme may have been due to peculiar characteristics about their setting, staff or participants. You are obliged to treat the imported programme as a whole new programme as soon as it is delivered to a new group of people by new staff. This means the same comprehensive process evaluation followed by the scaled-down monitoring programme once you are satisfied with you results.

What happens when you modify an existing programme to suit a new target group, like developing a package for non-English-speaking people? Again, you must treat this like a new programme. Your new group may react very differently. Your staff may adapt and change things as they go. Your programme materials may have cultural biases previously unrecognized.

A summary of the recommended level of process evaluation for programmes is given in Table 9.

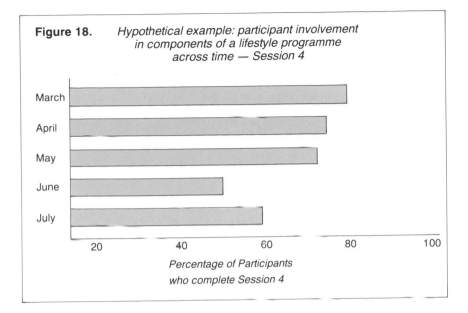

Figure 18.   *Hypothetical example: participant involvement in components of a lifestyle programme across time — Session 4*

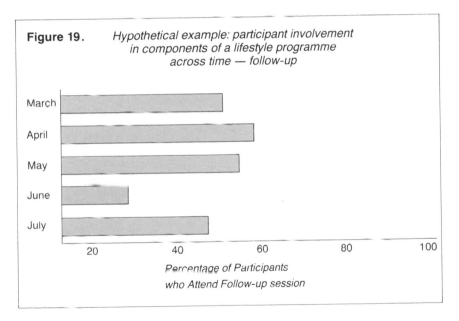

Figure 19.   *Hypothetical example: participant involvement in components of a lifestyle programme across time — follow-up*

Table 9. *How much process evaluation is recommended?*

Focus of Process Evaluation	Program Type	
	New programmes, imported programmes and programmes that obviously change in features such as target group, staff or methods and materials	Established programmes
1. Assessment of programme reach and proportion of components received by participants	Full range of techniques as appropriate until satisfied with results	Continuous
2. Assessment of participant satisfaction	Full range of techniques as appropriate until satisfied with results	Once every fouth time the programme is run but not less than once a year
3. Assessment of degree of programme implementation	Full range of techniques as appropriate until satisfied with results	Once every six sessions
4. Assessment of programme materials	Full range of techniques as appropriate until satisfied with results	Once every fouth time the programme is run but not less than once a year

Process Evaluation and Quality Assurance: What is Good Enough?

Our discussion so far has concentrated on getting your programme to an 'optimum level of functioning', collecting data and making changes to programmes until you are 'satisfied' with results or monitoring your programme to see if it continues to maintain the standard you might have set for programme reach or penetration into the target group. You may have wondered just what is good enough when it comes to the process of programme delivery and degree of implementation.

Remember that evaluation must involve both measurement and comparison of your observations to some criterion or standard. Unless you do this all you will have is research data and nothing to help you make decisions about programme performance—sooner or later the collection of data in this way will tire you, and chances are you will decide that evaluation is not worth the effort.

How do we solve the problem of standards or markers for good performance that we should try to reach? What are the standards? What is quality assurance?

It is not hard to find some definitions.

> Quality: *The appropriateness of a set of professional activities to the objectives they are attempting to achieve.*[7]

So we would all probably agree that a health promotion programme trying to use interpersonal communication, values clarification and peer support in order to reduce alcohol abuse in school children was more appropriate and therefore of better quality than a half-hour lecture trying to do the same thing.

> Quality assurance: *information provided that indicates that professional activities are being appropriately carried out.*[8]
> Quality control: *the actual surveillance system or procedures that are used to produce the information in quality assurance.*[7]

All the procedures and techniques we have so far outlined in process evaluation can be seen as quality control mechanisms to be used for quality assurance, provided that everyone knows what is an appropriate or not an appropriate activity in the first place. Unfortunately it is beyond the scope of this book to tell you what is the right or wrong way to design a specific programme to achieve a specific objective (we have pointed out already the relatively fail-safe general steps in programme planning to help you cover this). Our concern here is in the definition of 'appropriate' or 'good enough' or what is called the standard.

> Standard: *Minimum acceptable level of performance used to judge the quality of professional practice.*[11]

The hard part comes in quantifying this. Is a level of programme reach of 1 in 25 good enough? If 80% of participants complete the programme can we assume all is well? If 60% of women attending well baby clinics can understand your new leaflet should you go ahead and print 2000 copies? Unfortunately, specific advice in this areas is thin on the ground because health promotion is such a young field. It is very hard to be prescriptive because our experience is limited and people are loathe to make black and white performance indicators. There are moves in this direction but, meantime, we can tell you how to go about developing some reasonable standards or yardsticks that you can use.

Green and Lewis[9] have suggested that standards come from the following sources:

1. Historical comparisons with similar efforts in the past. So if you are in the field of immunization education and you are running a media

campaign you should try to get a level of target group awareness as good as or better than the data presented for the South Australian campaign in Table 6, page 62.

2. Comparisons with contemporary activities elsewhere. For example, if food hygiene leaflets produced by your state health department have readability scores of no greater than 12, then your new leaflet should have the same level or better.

3. Consensus among professionals, applying some combination of the first three.

Because data from process evaluations are often not published it may be hard to find comparative data. In this case you and your colleagues and supervisors must exercise some judgement and you must also canvass the opinions of others, in other areas. Often standards do not formally exist because the lack of process evaluation has meant that there has been no need for them to be clearly stated. The widespread development of routine process evaluation will contribute to the development and articulation of standards (which will of course vary with target group and programme strategy).

Summary and Conclusions

Process evaluation measures a programme's reach or penetration into the target group and the proportion of people in the group that receive all or only parts of your programme. Process evaluation also assesses the degree to which you have implemented your programme and your participants' satisfaction with it. Finally, process evaluation measures the quality of your programme materials, including the competencies of your staff. This information is used to improve your programme.

Comprehensive process evaluation is recommended for all new programmes as well as any programmes which have substantially changed or have been imported from another setting. When your process evaluation indicates that your programme is functioning in its optimum form, you can move on to impact and outcome evaluation. You must remember, though, to continue to do a scaled-down form of process evaluation to ensure that your programme is still running the way it should. Should your impact and outcome evaluation tell you that your programme works then the data from your process evaluation provides a clear documentation of what it is that works! Other people can then benefit by having all the information to set up your successful programme in their own areas. Congratulations!

References

1.   Weiss CM. *Evaluation research: methods for assessing program effectiveness*. Englewood Cliffs, NJ: Prentice-Hall, 1972.

2.   MacDonald H. Roder D. The planning, implementation and evaluation of an immunization promotion campaign in South Australia. *Hygie* 1985;4(2):13–17.

3.   US Department of Health and Human Services. National Cancer Institute. *Pretesting in health communications: methods, examples and resources for improving health message and materials.* NIH. Publication No. 81–1493. Washington DC: Government Printing Office, 1984.

4.   J. Miller and F. Lewis. Closing the Gap in Quality Assurance: A Tool for Evaluating Group Leaders. *Health Education Quarterly* 1982;9(1):55–66.

5.   Moos RH, Insel PM, Humphrey B. *Preliminary manual for family environment scale, work environment scale, group environment scale.* Palo Alto, California: Consulting Psychologists Press, 1974.

6.   Moos RH. *Evaluating Treatment Environment: A Social Ecological Approach.* New York: John Wiley and Sons, 1974.

7.   Windsor RA, Baranowski T, Clark N, Cutter G. *Evaluating Health Promotion and Health Education Programmes.* Palo Alto, California: Mayfield Publishing Company, 1984.

8.   Batey MV, Lewis FM. Clarifying autonomy and accountability in nursing service. Part 1. *Journal of Nursing Administration* 1982;12(9):13–18

9.   Green LW, Lewis FM. *Measurement and evaluation in health education and health promotion.* Palo Alto, California: Mayfield Publishing Company, 1986.

Further Reading

Windsor RA, Baranowski T, Clark N, Cutter G. *Evaluating Health Promotion and Health Education Programmes.* Palo Alto, California: Mayfield Publishing Company, 1984.

Chapter 5

EVALUABILITY ASSESSMENT: GETTING READY TO ASSESS PROGRAMME EFFECTS

OBJECTIVES

At the end of this chapter you should be able to:

1. Define evaluability assessment.
2. Identify those conditions that indicate that a programme is ready for impact and outcome evaluation.
3. Be able to apply the steps in evaluability assessment to your own programme.

What Does 'Evaluability Assessment' Mean?

Evaluability assessment is a term you will come across a lot as you read more about evaluation. What it refers to is the process you go through to make sure that a programme is ready for evaluation.[1,2] In other words, in evaluability assessment you check to see whether or not a programme satisfies a number of critical preconditions for evaluation. If these conditions are not satisfied you will run the risk of designing an impact or outcome evaluation which will collect inappropriate information about the programme. You also run the risk of conducting your evaluation prematurely—before the programme is likely to work. Evaluability assessment also makes you focus your attention on the sort of information about the programme performance that decision makers need. This makes sure that your evaluation produces usable data.

Strictly speaking, evaluability assessment refers to your review of the state of the programme at a particular point in time. However, in this chapter we are assuming that if you find the programme to be in an unfit state, you would want to rectify this. Therefore, when we talk about evaluability assessment here we will be referring to an active process of programme assessment and change, if change is required.

When you are satisifed with the results from your process evaluation that is, when you are satisfied with programme reach, participant satisfaction, implementation and quality, it is time to start thinking about how you will evaluate programme effects. There may be a range of interested parties who want to ask different questions about the programme. Most health promotion programmes are multifaceted, so there are many evaluation questions you could choose to address. Let's take, for example, a community-based cardiovascular disease prevention programme. Evaluation questions could be asked about the success of the programme in reducing the intake of dietary fat, or about reducing smoking, or in promoting exercise. Administrators may want to know if the screening vans are getting sufficient use, or should there be a return to hospital-based screening? Your community paediatrician may be suggesting that the first thing your evaluation should focus on is the impact on cholesterol levels in children.

There are decisions to make. These are about the focus of your evaluation, given that you won't have the resources to pursue all evaluation questions at once. You also have to make decisions about how you will conduct the evaluation, which measures you will use and so on. A major decision is whether your approach will be largely quantitative or qualitative. For example, do your decision makers require the type of evidence for programme effectiveness that can only be derived from a randomized controlled trial or will they be convinced by some case histories from people who have completed the programme? You will need to find out who needs information about the programme and whose needs are most urgent. In the example above is it the administrators wanting to know if it will be cheaper and as effective to do screening in the hospital or will you help your paediatrician, who is interested in the impact on different target groups?

Evaluability assessment provides a framework for making these decisions. It helps you to determine the shape of your evaluation. It also includes steps that have you rechecking programme implementation and programme rationale before you set out to examine programme effects. This is particularly important when you are evaluating an established programme or helping someone else evaluate a programme that you are not familiar with.

Why is there a Need for Evaluability Assessment?

If you have gone very carefully through the processes of needs assessment, programme planning and process evaluation, some of the common problems that evaluability assessment addresses will have been prevented. In the real world, however, impact and outcome evaluation does not always follow on from carefully conducted prior work. Consider the following situation.

Activity

Imagine that it is Heart Week and you are the area health promotion officer in a community health centre. Staff from the local hospital have organized a display at the local shopping centre. It consists of posters, pamphlets, a short video and a free blood pressure check. They ask you to design an evaluation for them that helps them to measure the blood pressure reduction in the community 12 months after the display. What would you do?

Feedback

As a skilled health educator you would probably know that the chances of this brief intervention having a substantial impact on the community's blood pressure levels are very low. This means that an evaluation designed to pick up this effect would probably be a waste of money. You have two choices. Either you persuade the staff to take an entirely new approach to blood pressure reduction programmes, or you evaluate their existing programme on more appropriate dimensions (say, focusing on changes in knowledge about salt intake and blood pressure).

The above situation focuses attention on a common situation in health promotion. Programmes are often poorly conceived and planned and this may not be apparent until evaluation plans begin. By recognizing the lack of fit between the activities of the blood pressure programme and its intended goals the health educator has addressed one aspect of evaluability assessment—making sure of the logic of the programme before designing an evaluation to assess programme effects.

For what other reasons is evaluability assessment needed? Consider the following.

Activity

Through successive changes of government in the past 7 years the community health programme in your state has had its staffing levels substantially reduced. Staffing levels are now at 65% of optimal level and a decision is to be made about whether to restore the programme. The present government wants to evaluate the current programme to determine whether claims that community health services promote health and reduce admissions to hospital can be justified. What do you think about the evaluation proposal?

Feedback

The evaluation is being put forward as an attempt to measure the effectiveness of community health before making decisions to restore the programme to its original optimal state. However, because the programme is not being adequately resourced at present it is extremely unlikely that any benefits of its preventive activities will be detected. If a programme is underresourced staff are usually diverted into a different range of activities addressing the most urgent needs and crises. If the evaluation goes ahead and finds minimal evidence of preventive success, decision makers may be led wrongly to conclude that the programme is incapable of achieving these effects.

The above is an example of what has been called a Type III error, which is evaluating something that does not really exist.[1] Unfortunately the mistake is rarely recognized and people are unaware of how wrong their conclusions about the programme may be. In evaluability assessment you make checks to ensure that the programme is properly implemented before you go looking for programme effects.

The final reason why evaluability assessment is needed is because many of the different groups associated with the programme may disagree about what the focus of the evaluation should be and what information should be collected. Often this problem does not become evident until the evaluation is complete and some groups ignore the results, or protest that the results are not useful. This has been called a Type IV error, evaluating something of no interest to decision makers.[1]

Some of the different interest groups might be administrators interested in costs and benefits, consumers who want to know about quality and outcome, and staff who may disagree about what components of the programme need to be addressed first. As part of the evaluability assessment you check with the different potential users of the information you will generate and get some agreement on what will be useful. By doing this before you start the evaluation proper you circumvent the risk that your data will not be relevant or of interest.

The 'Evaluable Programme': Preconditions for Evaluation

Premature or inappropriate evaluation of a programme is avoided by evaluability assessment. In evaluability assessment you check for a number of critical preconditions for evaluation. These mark the presence of what is called an 'evaluable programme', that is a programme in such a state that it can be evaluated meaningfully and usefully. These preconditions are:[1, 2]

1. There is a rational fit between clearly defined programme activities and the programme goals.

2. The programme is properly implemented.
3. There is agreement on what evaluation questions should be addressed.
4. There is agreement on how the evaluation should be conducted and what should be measured.

What happens if at first your programme does not appear to meet these preconditions? What happens if a programme is not evaluable? The answer is that you don't proceed with the evaluation. Instead you spend time in programme redesign and planning, administration and management and in talking with the various groups involved with the programme until the preconditions for evaluation are fulfilled. Then you proceed with the evaluation. What follows now is a step-by-step guide in evaluability assessment which will help you to identify what is happening with a programme and rectify any shortfalls in the fulfilment of preconditions for evaluation.

Steps in Evaluability Assessment

Step 1—Identify the primary users of the evaluation information. Find out what they need to know.

Activity
Imagine that a preparation for parenthood programme has been running for a number of years at an infant welfare clinic. An evaluation of the programme is now proposed. Can you identify the different groups who might want to know about the programme's performance? What type of information might they require? Make a brief list.

Feedback
A range of people may be interested and this is significant because they all might have different views or opinions about what sort of evaluation information should be collected. The group might include infant welfare staff, hospital maternity ward staff, local general practitioners, community health centre staff, the Nursing Mothers Association and administrators of your funding authorities. The range of evaluation questions might include: 'Does the programme reduce birth complications?' 'Does the programme increase breast feeding?' 'Are parents less anxious about parenting as a result of the programme?' 'In the child's first year does the programme reduce visits to doctors for minor illnesses or trouble?' 'Does the programme provide a better form of antenatal care and education than parents can get from their own doctors?' 'Is it as good as but cheaper than traditional care?'

The type of evaluation study you need to design to see if a programme improves breast feeding practices is considerably simpler than one you would need to design to assess and compare the costs and effectiveness of different forms of antenatal care. As evaluation resources are scarce you don't want to put yourself in the situation of collecting too much information. Neither do you want to collect insufficient or the wrong sort of information. This is why you need to decide who the primary users of your evaluation will be and what their information needs are and cater your study to them. These are likely to be the people who will make decisions about the programme. If your primary users are administrators or funding authorities, they will probably be making decisions about maintaining or extending the programme. If your primary users are colleagues or other agencies, they may be making decisions about referring people to your programme.

A good way to approach this issue is to ask your users, the intended audience of your evaluation, a direct question like: 'What would my programme need to demonstrate for you to continue funding it?' or 'What sorts of changes or improvements would you like to see among the people attending this programme for you to start sending people along?'

Remember, however, that a single evaluation study could not hope to answer all the evaluation questions about a programme, particularly as health promotion programmes are often so complex and multifaceted. You may have to discuss these things with your intended users and put questions into priority order. Remember too that some expectations held about a programme may not be realistic. It is up to you to educate and sensitize your users as well as listen to their needs. Once the main audience for your evaluation is known and the main evaluation questions are identified, your evaluation plans may begin to take shape.

Step 2 — Define the programme

This may sound a little obvious, but as part of the evaluability assessment you need to be sure that you can really define what the programme is and sometimes this is hard. For example, say after each weight control group you run it takes about half an hour or so before you can close up the room because people are standing around chatting. Is this half hour part of the programme? Does it contribute to programme goals? It might, if you're are trying to foster social contact. You can see that distinguishing what is 'programme' from what is merely part of the background activity or general running of the organization or centre is not as easy as it first seems.

A useful strategy is to ask programme staff to define the programme in such a way that would allow others to reproduce it. Encourage people to define the programme boundaries. Make sure that you talk to all the people involved in running the programme because you may be surprised to find that people describe the programme differently. You may need to get them all together to get some consensus on what is and what isn't the programme. This is essential to your evaluation because when you show effects people will want to know what it was that caused them! If you have already conducted a full process evaluation of the programme this step should be relatively easy.

Step 3 — Specify goals and expected effects

The programme plan should have within it clearly defined goals, but a programme may have escaped this step. Maybe you are helping someone else with their evaluation and the programme goals are only stated generally. Maybe goal specification seemed too hard!

For a goal to be amenable to evaluation, things must be stated in terms of time, person, place and amount. It is insufficient to say: 'To reduce the number of children admitted to hospital for asthma'. You must be more specific, for example 'To reduce the number of admissions to hospital for asthma in children aged 10 to 16 years by 25% by the end of 1995'. With a goal this clearly spelt out any person could examine hospital records in 1996 and recognize whether or not the programme's goal had been achieved. Further, unless you do specify the amount of change desired a statistician cannot tell you how many people you will need in your study to test if your programme has achieved this change. This is something we will talk about again in Chapter 6.

How do you get people to be so specific, particularly about how much change they want to see achieved? Again you may need to be very direct with people to help them to articulate their performance standards. Would a 30% reduction in asthma admissions be a success? Why? Would a 5% reduction in asthma admissions be a success? Why not?

Where do these numbers come from? These are the criteria by which you judge the performance of your programme. Your consideration of these is a critical factor in your evaluation. To try to find a performance standard you should first look at the normal expected fluctuations in the factor of interest. For example, if asthma admissions each year seem to go up or down by about 5% you would certainly want to see a bigger reduction achieved as a result of the implementation of your programme. So to get started you should gather these data together and give programme staff or the users of your evaluation a picture of what usually happens. Any seasonal fluctuations should also be noted as this might affect not only when you should time the introduction of your programme but also how you might interpret your results.

Another consideration in setting your performance standard is the success other people might have achieved from similar programmes. For example, if other asthma education programmes achieved reductions in hospital admission rates in the order of 15% to 20% you should aim to do at least as well, or better.

When the epidemiology of a disease is well known, mathematical modelling may help you set the performance standard in your goal. For example, with a highly infectious disease such as measles it has been suggested that we need to get upwards of 95% of all children vaccinated. However with smallpox, which is a less infectious disease, a smaller proportion of the population needed to be vaccinated for the disease to be eradicated. [3]

So much for the goals of the programme, what about other effects? A number of authorities on evaluation have pointed out the importance of looking at both intended and unintended effects of a programme. [4] The intended effects are usually the goals but the unintended effects can have considerable consequence. For example, often whenever we set up a health promotion programme we are interested in prevention and we set out to reach a proportion of the population perhaps hitherto not involved with the health services. As a result of this we may uncover undetected problems. For example, people attending a health screening checkpoint at a health fair may hear of the community health service for the first time. Increases in referrals to the centre may put such a pressure of workload on staff that the activity of the original health promotion programme may need to be curtailed. In evaluability assessment, these possibilities must be anticipated so that your evaluation is designed to pick up all likely effects, whether goal-linked or not.

Step 4 — Ensure that causal assumptions in the programme are plausible

Activity
You are helping some colleagues prepare to evaluate a programme that is trying to prevent school children experimenting with and subsequently continuing to take illegal drugs. The programme consists of a mobile display taken through schools and recreation centres that depicts illegal drugs and lists the health and social consequences of drug use. It has many photographs and histories of young drug users and is accompanied by an ex-addict who talks to school groups about the danger of drug use. How would you determine that this strategy is likely to achieve the desired goal of preventing drug use?

Feedback
Firstly you would talk to programme staff and consult programme plans to determine their analysis of the health problem of interest (why

kids experiment and take up drugs) and why it is thought that this particular strategy should prevent this occurring. It would be appropriate to determine the models or theories of health promotion or health or social behaviour that support this view. You should look for the existence of evidence that supports the strategy chosen, i.e., the documented success of this strategy in other situations. Alternatively, if no evidence supports the venture, or if there is evidence to the contrary, a critical review of other drug education strategies should be undertaken to justify what the designers of the programme are proposing to undertake.

A lot of this work should have been completed as part of the programme planning and therefore should not be difficult to retrieve. However, if you are doing evaluability assessment with a programme that does not have this documentation then the situation is more difficult. Whose job is it to go back to the stage of literature review for the justification of programme rationale? If it is your own programme then it is your job to do the work that justifies the selection of programme strategies and thereby spells out the programme's caual thinking. If you are helping with the evaluation of a programme that is not your own, then this point can be quite uncomfortable and explains why evaluation is sometimes seen as threatening! No one likes to be told that they need to go back over things but the consequences of not doing so are too great. It is far better to guide people into rethinking and redesigning their programme if necessary than to ignore this and conduct an evaluation that shows that their programme doesn't work. Then they really won't like you!

Even if you are only helping someone else with the evaluation of a programme it is worth familiarizing yourself with the literature or background material to the programme plan. This helps you to discuss things more easily with programme staff. In fact, rechecking programme rationale prior to impact or outcome evaluation can be made into an invigorating 'time out' or 'think tank'. Often a dip back into the current literature about programmes similar to yours can provide new support for the programme rationale. People can get a better or different perspective on their programme and its possible contribution to the health problem of interest. Alternatively, you may decide to take on some new features in the light of what you read and assess. This will of course delay subsequent impact or outcome evaluation because you will first need to rerun your process evaluation to see how well any new programme features fit in with your staff and participants. This is an illustration of how evaluability assessment contributes to programme development.

Step 5 — Reach agreement on measurable and testable programme activities and goals

In process evaluation you would have racked your brains to come up with ways to monitor or record what went on in your programme. You would have devised measures for programme attendance, session content and so on. This is all to ensure that your programme activities are measurable and therefore verifiable in some objective sense.

You may not have devised ways to measure all aspects of the programme. For example, in the feedback forms you get back from participants a number of people may say how good it was when they were enrolling in the programme to have such a friendly and interested person receiving their calls and answering their questions. Having a friendly, warm receptionist in your outpatients clinic might be a real plus. However, you may not consider this such an important item that you ask all participants to rate their conversation with the receptionist as 'warm, neutral or cold' and start talking about the proportion of warm encounters and so on! Measurement on this scale may be taking things a little too far. In this phase of evaluability assessment you reach some agreement with the users or audience for your evaluation about what is the best way to measure and record programme activity. You work out what's worth monitoring and what is not.

In this step you also have to make a decision about the way in which you are going to measure the achievement of programme goals. For example, the regional coordinator of children's health services and yourself may have decided that in your evaluation of an asthma education programme you should see if the programme increases compliance with asthma medications, reduces wheezing episodes and reduces asthma-related doctor consultations and hospital admissions. All of these things therefore must be measured and you and your regional coordinator must agree on the way this should be done because differences might arise in the quality or standard of evidence. For example, compliance with asthma medications might be measured by a questionnaire. However, some people might be more convinced if a more objective measure was used—for example, weighing and counting of medications left in a bottle at the conclusion of a time period (thereby allowing the proportion actually taken to be calculated). Similarly, you could ask parents the number of times they had taken their child to see a doctor for an asthma-related complaint over a 3-month period or you could rely on records kept by the medical practice.

Ultimately, when you conclude that a programme has improved medication compliance or reduced the need for emergency care you don't want the potential users of your information to dispute the quality of your measures. That is why you need to agree on the measures to be used before you start.

In this step of evaluability assessment, you also need to consider the possibility that not all the programme goals are going to be measurable and able to be tested. For example, another facet of your asthma education programme may have been to try to tackle the problem of children using their illness to seek attention in the family and win favours or concessions over their brothers or sisters. How can such a thing be measured? How would you know whether or not such a goal had been achieved? You may 'draw a blank' on some goals and never feel that you can devise a satisfactory form of measurement.

First of all take some time to see what other people think, especially people working full-time in evaluation, research or health planning units in health departments or tertiary institutions. These people have the advantage of being able to monitor the literature on the development of new instruments to measure such things as social support, community identity or competence, or the value people place on health. Secondly, if you really can't generate any helpful suggestions then try not to worry too much about it. Health promotion is a rapidly developing and creative field. Sometimes innovation in evaluation may have to lag a little behind! We hope, however, that this doesn't happen too often or we may end up only being able to prove that health promotion makes an impact on relatively run-of-the-mill things while our more exciting but abstract achievements go uncelebrated!

Step 6 — Reach agreement on what is sufficient in the evaluation

By this stage in your evaluability assessment you may have found the need to scale down and narrow the original focus on what the evaluation should demonstrate. You now need to make sure that what you are able to do is sufficient to answer worthwhile questions about the programme and supply decision makers with information to help them determine what happens next.

In our experience, a good way to help people to appreciate what an evaluation will and will not show is to make up dummy tables, graphs and illustrations of what your results could show. By 'dummy' tables we mean tables that show the title and dimensions of your data but for which the actual data or results are missing or fictitious. For example, titles of tables might be 'Smoking rates by age group' or 'Smoking rates of people who attended less than half the programme sessions'. 'Of those who had previously tried to quit smoking – reason given for failing to quit in this programme'. These give quick impressions of the nature and intricacies of the data you are about to produce. Any omissions are obvious and if appropriate these evaluation questions can be included to correct them.

Step 7 — Make sure that the programme is being implemented as intended

Finally you need to check to make sure that the programme really is up and running the way it should be. The chapter on process evaluation illustrates some of the techniques you might use. The reason for this assessment or reassessment prior to impact or outcome evaluation is to make sure that the programme is given its best chance to work by having optimum levels of implementation. Only when a programme is fully implemented do you have the opportunity to test whether the combination of programme strategies that you have chosen leads to the changes in health knowledge, attitude, behaviour or any other set of factors of concern to you.

What happens if you find that in spite of everything you try, there is drop out from the programme? In other words if not all the programme components are received by all programme participants, what then? Is it possible to still look at programme effects? The answer is a cautious 'yes', provided that (1) after further attempts you are confident that implementation and the proportion of programme components received by participants cannot be improved and (2) that a sufficiently large number of people receive all the programme components in a satisfactory form. You must, however, also look at programme effects separately for each subgroup of participants that received different exposure to your programme.

Consider, for example, a weight control programme. Of all those who enrolled in your programme at Week 1, let's say that 65% had attained their personal ideal goal weight 10 weeks later. By referring to the success rate as a percentage of all people enrolled this figure acknowledges the fact that attendance at such a programme was less than ideal and that a lot of people might not have attended the later sessions nor followed a home maintenance plan. So this figure of 65% success includes consideration of some of the real-life problems in programme implementation and is a realistic overall figure to quote about the programme to others who might wish to duplicate it. However, within your group there may be some people who attended all sessions and followed the home maintenance plan. The success rate for this group may be 85%. Also within the group there may have been those who tiring of your regimen and not liking the group dropped out after session 2. Your programme's success rate for this group may have been only 15%. Analysing your data in this way may give you some of the extra inspiration needed to devise ways to keep people in the programme!

The above example illustrates the difference between two terms used in programme evaluation. One is 'efficacy', which refers to how great the benefit of an intervention is shown to be under optimal conditions (e.g. optimum programme implementation). The other is 'effectiveness', which refers to how great the benefit of an intervention is shown to be in practice (e.g. with the reality of incomplete attendance, etc.). In the example we have given the figure of 65% refers to the programme's effectiveness, while the figure 85% demonstrates programme efficacy. The gap between the two can be narrowed as effort is made to make the operations and implementation of the programme as close as possible to the ideal intended.

Table 10. *Evaluability assessment of a patient medication education programme (summary)*

STEPS IN EVALUABILITY ASSESSMENT

Programme description	Programme goals	1. Identify primary users of the evaluation. Find out what they need to know.	2. Articulate the programme.	3. Specify goals and expected effects.	4. Ensure causal assumptions are plausible.	5. Reach agreement on measurable and testable programme activities and goals	6. Reach agreement on what is sufficient in the evaluation.	7. Ensure that programme is implemented as intended.
Programme consists of two one-hour talks about taking medications led by a pharmacist to a group of patients on a hospital ward.	1. To improve medication compliance (proportion of patients who take correct amount of medications). 2. To reduce consumption of over the counter medications. 3. To improve self-responsibility in relation to the patient's health.	Health department funding committee for patient education in hospital. Questions: Does programme improve compliance? Does programme reduce hospital admissions for drug-related disorders?	Talking to staff and attending sessions reveals that programme consists of: 1. Two group sessions each about 60 minutes — 6 topics: names/ strengths of drugs; directions on label; interactions/ allergies; storage; how to use medication card; over the counter medications.	1. To reduce over-dosage (taking more than 120% of recommended dose) by 15%. 2. To reduce underdosage (taking less than 80% of recommended dose) by 15%. 3. To reduce taking of old medications by 15%. 4. To reduce taking of other people's medications by 15%.	1. Group education sessions with individual follow-up personal counselling with own medication card tailored to patients is a strategy likely to work e.g. Mullen et al *Preventive Medicine* 1985; 14(6):753–781. 2. However, such little time is spent on discussion of over the counter medications	1. Content of sessions can be monitored by an observer. 2. Time devoted to counselling can be monitored by a pharmacist. 3. Medication cards received and used by patients can be monitored by questionnaire. 4. Drug compliance goals can be meas-	Programme staff contact Regional health advisors to discuss the proposal. Programme Funding Committee reviews the formal evaluation proposal and agrees to it.	Attendance at the session usually held one week later is poor, often because patients have been discharged. Resolved to abandon second session and improve quality and content of the first session. Other educators have had success with a single session e.g. Wandless and Davie *British*

Average number of patients is 9 per week.

2. Personal counselling after the session by a pharmacist for about 15 minutes with each patient.

3. Personalised medication record card to be carried by patient at all times to help patient and prescribing doctors.

Degree of reduction desired in the 12-week period post discharge follows report of Macdonald et al *British Medical Journal* 1977; 2:613–621.

that this goal should be dropped. This will allow more session time to be spent on drug compliance goals.

ured by questionnaire after testing that this is as good as counting up pills left in bottles and deducing compliance this way.

5. Goal regarding self-responsibility for health cannot be specified and measured satisfactorily.

6. Drug-related hospital admissions can only be satisfactorily assessed at hospital running the programme. Admissions to other hospitals will be difficult to track down.

Medical Journal 1977; 1:359–361.

Summary and Conclusions

Table 10 is an illustration of the steps in evaluability assessment applied to a patient education programme. You can see that as you read the columns from left to right the shape of the programme and its goals becomes much more specific, tangible and evaluable.

Writers in evaluability assessment refer to two models or two versions of what a programme is and does. These are the 'rhetorical programme model' or what staff and documents say the programme is, and the 'evaluable programme model' which is what is left out of the rhetorical programme model after the unmeasurable objectives, unmeasurable or non-existent activities, weak rationale and unstable assumptions have been elimated![2] This may sound a little harsh. However, increasing rigor in health promotion planning and practice means that few health promotion programmes these days would be demolished by evaluability assessment. Rather, the process can enhance and develop programmes into a form where they are most likely to demonstrate their worth. Because the time and resources that go into evaluation of programme effects (impact and outcome evaluation) are quite extensive, the opportunity to evaluate effects of a programme rarely arises more than once or twice. When the time comes you want to make sure that your programme is truly ready. This is why every step in evaluability assessment must be considered with care.

References

1. Scanlon JW, Horst P, Jay JN, Schmidt RE, Waller JD. Evaluability assessment: avoiding Type III and Type IV errors. In Gilbert GR, Conklin PJ (eds) *Evaluation Management: A source book of readings* Charlottesville: US Civil Service Commission, 1977.
2. Wholey JS. Evaluability assessment. In Rutman L (ed). *Evaluative Research Methods: A Basic Guide* Beverly Hills; Sage Publications, 1977.
3. Anderson RM, May RM. Vaccination and herd immunity to infectious diseases. *Nature* 1985:318:323–329.
4. Scriven, M. Pros and cons of goal-free evaluation. *Evaluation Comment* 1972;3(4):–7.

Chapter 6
IMPACT AND OUTCOME EVALUATION: ASSESSING PROGRAMME EFFECTS

OBJECTIVES

At the end of this chapter you should be able to:

1. Explain the difference between impact and outcome evaluation.
2. Time your impact or outcome evaluation to coincide with when you expect effects to occur.
3. Determine which aspects of your approach to assessing programme effects will be qualitative and which will be quantitative.
4. Choose your approach to measuring changes in knowledge, attitude, behaviour, health status, social support, quality of life, health costs, community cohesion and competence.
5. Design a pre-test and post-test (or 'before and after') evaluation for your programme.
6. Write a report to convey your methods and findings.

By the end of evaluability assessment you should have a very specific question (or questions) about programme performance. You may want to know, for example, if your programme reduces unnecessary hospital admissions for the elderly, or improves parents' knowledge about childhood asthma or leads to the development of social support networks among young families in new housing estates. You now have to start thinking more carefully about what it is you wish to measure. You also have to start thinking about when you feel the programme's effects should be evident. Also, can you really be sure that you will be able to conclude that the programme, rather than some other factor or event, caused the effects you see? Just how sophisticated will your evaluation design have to be to sort out the influence of these other factors? What will this mean in terms of additional resources? These are the issues we will address in this chapter.

What is the Difference between Impact and Outcome Evaluation?

Impact and outcome evaluation both involve the assessment of programme effects but at different levels. Impact evaluation is concerned with the assessment of the immediate effects of the programme and usually corresponds with the measurement of the programme objective. Outcome evaluation is concerned with the subsequent or longer-term effects of the programme and this usually corresponds to the programme goal. For example, a cardiac rehabilitation programme might be attempting to improve the exercise and dietary habits of people admitted with their first heart attack, with the goal of reducing the likelihood of subsequent attacks. Impact evaluation would assess changes in dietary and exercise habits and outcome evaluation would assess the incidence of subsequent heart attacks.

Activity
A community worker is trying to set up social support networks among new mothers in the hope that this will help reduce the incidence of loneliness and depression among them. What would the impact evaluation of this programme measure? What would the outcome evaluation of this programme measure?

Feedback
The impact evaluation would assess the changes made in social support (that is, did social support increase?). The outcome evaluation would assess the change made to the prevalence of depression.

Activity
A youth worker is attempting to improve community awareness about the plight of homeless youth in the hope of encouraging community action and support to set up a youth refuge. What would the impact evaluation measure? What would outcome evaluation measure?

Feedback
Impact evaluation would assess community awareness and attitudes towards homeless youth (did the intervention increase community

awareness and concern?). Outcome evaluation would assess community support and action (however defined: for example, community fund raising, setting up of committee structures, putting together of a submission, etc.).

You can see that impact and outcome evaluation tests the theory or causal chain of events that has been postulated by the programme. For example, that changing knowledge will lead to a change in behaviour or that improving social support will reduce stress-related conditions. This comes from your analysis of the health problem and the factors contributing to it which you considered in the second stage of needs assessment and which you set out to address in your programme plan.

However, like your programme planning strategies, what you measure in impact and outcome evaluation depends very much on where you sit in the health system. Remember that one person's objective can be another person's goal. So with impact and outcome evaluation you may be assessing one factor in outcome evaluation, while another person may be assessing the same factor as part of their impact evaluation. This is why we are dealing with both impact and outcome evaluation in the same chapter.

For example, at an area level, a health educator may be trying to affect a change in knowledge and attitudes about nutrition (impact evaluation) with the goal of improving dietary habits (outcome evaluation). On a state or national level planners and researchers may be assessing changes in dietary habits (impact evaluation) with the goal of reducing the incidence of cardiovascular disease (outcome evaluation).

So, the difference between impact and outcome evaluation does not depend on what is measured, but it is defined by the sequence of measurement. This means that you cannot say just by looking at a factor whether it should be measured in impact evaluation or whether it should be measured in outcome evaluation. It depends entirely on the causal chain of events that has been postulated and where each programme stands in relation to these. Many individual programmes run in areas or states may add up to a national strategy with one effect leading to another. If, for example, we limited ourselves to thinking that all goals had to be stated in terms of health status (as some texts suggest) then this would mean that only those health workers working at a level in the health system where they are sufficiently resourced to measure these changes (usually at regional, state or national levels) would conduct outcome evaluation. All other health workers would be 'let off the hook'.

Why would this be so terrible? Because if many programmes were restricted to the assessment of impact only, programme 'success' would tend to become too narrowly and prematurely defined; that is, it would be confined to the achievement of immediate objectives. These objectives might cover things such as knowledge, awareness, attitudes and so on. While theory in health promotion is still being developed and tested, we cannot be sure that changes in these factors will ultimately guarantee changes in health status at some point 'higher up the line'. We are obliged, therefore, to encourage the people responsible for programmes at all levels to follow through their bit of the causal chain and measure immediate effects (impact) and subsequent effects (outcome) no matter what factors they actually measure at each point.

Is it always possible to define the causal chain of events or the expected sequence of factors for impact and outcome evaluation? This depends on your model or stategy. With educational approaches most health educators would venture to suppose that they have to influence attitudes or knowledge and skills before they can bring about behaviour change. Evaluations subsequently determine when the theory does or does not hold, say when sufficient evidence was accumulated to demonstrate that knowledge alone is an insufficient precursor for behaviour change.[1]

With other approaches, events might not be so easy to predict and this affects evaluation planning. For example, in community development many people would argue that it is impossible to say in which direction a community will proceed when they set out to tackle health issues or problems, so this cannot be specified in programme goals. Many effects may also go undetected because they were not suspected beforehand and information was not sought.

There are ways to tackle this. Firstly, in relation to the latter problem, unstructured qualitative investigations can discover effects and repercussions and these are the subject of discussion later in this chapter. In relation to the first problem, your evaluation approach will depend entirely on what you see the role of community development in health to be. So again it relates to theory and philosophy. With some approaches, impact and outcome evaluation will be focused on what you (or perhaps rather, your community) consider success to be and how it will be brought about. It could be changes in the community lobbying and decison making power as might be evidenced in the formation of action groups, winning resources, perceived power and community self-confidence, shared community perspectives, concern for local issues and so on. Alternatively, you may consider community involvement more as an indicator of quality programme process (so it is measured in process evaluation) and your impact and outcome evaluation would proceed in a similar vain to other more traditional models; that is, it might be focused on achievement of changes in health knowledge, attitudes, behaviours and so on. We cannot tell you exactly what to evaluate in impact and outcome evaluation. This is your decision based on your model, philosophy and strategy. However, designing your impact and outcome evaluation will force you to address the thinking and principles behind the intervention you have designed.

How to Measure Programme Effects

Programmes in health promotion, health education and patient education cover a diversity of topic areas and target groups. The intention of many programmes is to bring about change in preventive health behaviour such as seat belt use, parenting, sexual behaviour and so on. Programmes may also be directed at making changes at environmental or societal levels. These might include changes in the food supply or immunization laws or the allocation of public space to no smoking zones or changes in social networks. Some programmes are simply trying to improve the skills of the community itself in dealing with the health problems and issues that affect the community.

How do you measure changes in these areas? In this section we demonstrate some approaches to the measurement of changes in some common areas. These changes may be in the areas covered by your programme objectives and programme goals, but they may also include changes outside these areas, so-called unintended effects.

Qualitative and quantitative methods of investigation

The way in which you set out to investigate programme effects can be divided into two distinct approaches. These are qualitative approaches and quantitative approaches. Qualitative methods describe approaches where you seek to interpret the meaning of the programme for programme participants, programme staff and also people not reached by the programme. The methods are largely unstructured and observational. This contrasts with quantitative methods where you have a notion of what effects you wish to detect and you set out to measure these systematically, using standardized measuring instruments and then scoring these measures and subjecting them to quantitative manipulation. Some people like to summarize this by saying that qualitative approaches answer questions to do with the 'why' of a programme while quantitative approaches look at 'how much'; qualitative methods subsequently lead to the analysis of words and meanings and quantitative methods lead to the analysis of numbers.

Both approaches have strengths. Qualitative approaches are particularly good for finding out about unintended effects and for understanding why effects (both intended and unintended) occured. As is discussed in later chapters, you use open-ended questions, such as 'What do you think (the programme) did for people in (this area)?' To find out why certain things happened, you go out and ask people. This gives you a greater understanding of the effect of your programme. Let's take the result: 'Only 3% of participants changed their exercise habits'. Without a qualitative investigation you may not be able to learn why this happened.

The strength of quantitative methods is that their standard, systematic and usually much briefer approach allows you to reach more people in your investigation and make comparisons among them. Usually, the dimensions covered in quantitative measures, say scales to measure depression or health status, come from what has been discovered from qualitative approaches, that is from people going out and asking people about their experiences. With quantitative approaches you can measure the size of an effect.

Both approaches have limitations. In qualitative approaches, a large amount of 'in depth' data is gathered from, say, people connected with the programme, but this may mean that only relatively few people can be interviewed and it is hard to generalize the findings. With quantitative approaches, data can be fairly easily collected from a large number of people, but the depth and detail of differences in experiences is sacrificed.

In both evaluation and needs assessment you probably will use both types of approaches to interpret what is happening, and a lot of this is also tied to the stage of your evaluation and the type of information you need to acquire. In the early stages of a new programme, you may need to rely more on qualititative methods to develop a sense about the range of effects that may have occured. With an established programme, effects may be more familiar and your interest may be to assess their magnitude. Chapter 7 has a section on analysis of qualitative and quantitative data.

So, if your approach is to be entirely unstructured and open ended you will go out looking for all sorts of effects, whether they are related to the programme goals or not. This is termed 'goal-free' evaluation.[2] However, chances are you already have a notion about what it is you will want to measure and this will have come out of your evaluability assessment. This can be pursued using both qualitative and quantitative methods and you will have to make some decisions about this depending perhaps on the type of information you want to collect and your own judgement about what is appropriate.

For example, in trying to understand the effect of a support programme for adolescent victims of domestic violence, you might interview all participants in a fairly unstructured way to become sensitized to the range of effects the programme might have had. However, if you were evaluating the effectiveness of such programmes across the state, you might subsequently opt to use a self-administered self-esteem measure.

There may be occasions when you conclude that a standardized measuring instrument or quantitative approach might never truly capture a programme's effects. The meaning of the programme and the experience of the effects by participants might not be able to be summarized in a score on a 60-item questionnaire. There also may be occasions when you opt for a standardized measure because you might consider an unstructured interview-based approach to be too intrusive or inappropriate.

We suggest that, once you have decided what you want to measure and how you will approach this, you should check to see if any other investigators have published their instruments or measures before you set out to design your own. Using their measures will make your job easier and allow you to compare your data directly with theirs. You should consult the chapters on how to choose a measure and questionnaire design. If you are going to use an entirely qualitative approach you may also decide to seek some advice on how to do this (see Chapter 11).

The section that follows outlines some important considerations in relation to some common impacts and outcomes in health promotion. This may help to focus your thinking when you are selecting a measure or designing your own.

Measuring knowledge

This is where you attempt to assess what people know, what people recognize or what they are aware of, what they understand and what people have learned. Your approach to each of these may vary.

Activity

You are interested in assessing community awareness of a skin cancer prevention campaign and you have decided to survey people in shopping centres. What sort of question would you ask people?

Feedback

A common way to do this is to approach people and ask: 'Are you aware of the skin cancer prevention campaign that is being run at the present time?' or 'Have you seen or heard any of the recent publicity about skin cancer prevention?' However, the problem with the way these questions are phrased is that respondents are likely to say 'Yes' because they may have realized that you want them to! This is termed a 'demand characteristic' in the question. A better way to determine the true extent of public awareness would be to present to people a list of a number of different campaigns (real or fictitious) and place your skin cancer campaign somewhere on this list. Show them the list and ask them about their awareness of each campaign in turn. Then it is difficult for respondents to guess your interests and they are more likely to give you true answers. Don't make the list too long, however, as you will risk tiring or annoying respondents before you get to the item of real interest.

Note that this technique merely gives you information on campaign awareness. This is a prequisite to anything else (unless you are into subliminal approaches!), but it may not be sufficient for your needs. You don't know as yet what they have learned from exposure to your campaign, but the technique is good for sorting out groups with whom you may pursue a further line of questioning.

Activity
How would you assess what people have learned from your campaign?

Feedback
Unless people have agreed to be explicitly involved in a learning situation such as in a training course or education group, you will probably find that they do not react well to the question: 'What did you learn?', simply because a lot of people like to think that they don't have to be 'taught' anything. Your campaign may also not reflect this style of approach. It may be better to ask 'What did the campaign tell people to do to prevent skin cancer?' Note here, however, that what the question is really addressing is recall of the campaign message. This may not necessarily equate with comprehension. To assess comprehension you can set up a question that requires the respondent to use the information he or she has learned and apply it to some problem. For example, rather that asking people to recall the content of messages in a nutrition campaign, you can ask them to pick out from a list the food item with the least fat content.

What about assessment of knowledge in those situations where people are part of an education or training programme? In these situations people have wittingly placed themselves in a learning or training mode and you can probably ask them to complete a self-administered questionnaire. For example, you may have respondents read statements about a particular topic and have them indicate which statements they feel are true or false. Another format is the multiple choice format where respondents select the 'correct' answer from a series of alternatives.

An example would be:

please tick only one answer

To reduce your cholesterol level you should
- a. give up salt   [ ]
- b. eat less fat   [√]
- c. eat less bread   [ ]

More examples of question formats are given in Chapter 7 in the section on questionnaire design. Finally, you should beware of approaches that ask people to rate their knowledge about a subject at the beginning of a programme and then ask them to rate their knowledge at the end of the programme. This is because what may change as a result of the programme may not simply be their knowledge but also their beliefs about the size and scope of the subject. So, for example, health workers attending a training course on AIDS at the beginning may rate their knowledge on the subjects as 'very good', but at the end of the programme they may rate their knowledge as 'good', even if they have learnt a lot more. The apparent lack of progress may simply reflect the fact that at the end of the programme they may be more fully aware of the complexity of the AIDS area and they now have become more modest in their self-assessment.

Measuring attitudes

Measuring attitudes is a little trickier than measuring knowledge because how people feel about something is a little harder to pin down in black and white. You need to encourage more freedom in expression and you may find, particularly when you first set out to explore an issue, that qualitative methods offer the most assistance.

Activity

You are evaluating a programme which has as its goal the prevention of alcohol abuse and drink driving among adolescents. Part of the programme involves trying to reverse the traditional stereotype that associates having a good time with alcohol. The objective is to promote positive attitudes about alcohol-free recreation and socializing. In your impact evaluation you want to assess adolescents' views about drinking and fun, drinking and parties, drinking and sport and so on. How would you do this?

Feedback

There are a number of techniques you can choose from. A useful approach would be to show small groups of adolescents short videos depicting adolescents refusing alcohol and socializing without alcohol and asking them questions like: 'What do you think of this girl?' 'What do you think her friends think of her?' and so on. See also Chapter 9 on how to run a focus group. With larger groups of adolescents you could use a questionnaire, such as the one that is illustrated in Table 11 which gets respondents to indicate their feelings about a range of statements. (See also Chapter 7.)

Measuring behaviour

On many occasions the purpose of the health promotion programme is to bring about a change in people's health or preventive health behaviour. We might want them to eat more nutritious foods, or exercise more or immunize their children or stay out of the sun in the middle of the day or simply talk and get to know their neighbours. How do you know whether behaviour change has occurred?

The simplest thing to do is to ask them! That is, your measure of behaviour can be self-report. For example, in the evaluation of the

Table 11. *Measuring attitudes*

*Please circle the number that most closely matches
how you feel about each statement*

If you often get really drunk your friends don't respect you.	Strongly Agree 1_____	Agree 2_____	Don't Know 3_____	Disagree 4_____	Strongly Disagree 5
You can't have fun at a party without alcohol.	Strongly Agree 1_____	Agree 2_____	Don't Know 3_____	Disagree 4_____	Strongly Disagree 5
I would be embarrassed to refuse a drink at a party when everyone else was drinking.	Strongly Agree 1_____	Agree 2_____	Don't Know 3_____	Disagree 4_____	Strongly Disagree 5

Sydney 'Quit. For Life.' anti-smoking campaign, interviewers asked people whether they were a 'smoker', an 'ex-smoker' or a person who had never smoked.[3] Fortunately it has been shown that this is a valid measure of smoking status.[4] That is, self-report of behaviour in relation to this question is likely to give accurate results.

However, with other questions and in other sorts of topic areas the replies are likely to be less accurate. For example, researchers in Newcastle found that parents do not accurately report their use of child safety restraints in cars. Many more parents report using restraints than the proportion of parents actually observed if you stand outside kindergartens and watch what happens.[5] Similarly, if you try to assess the proportion of children in the community that have been immunized against measles, you will find that interviews with parents will give you higher estimates than if you used a more accurate measure such as analysis of childrens' blood samples.[6]

Generally speaking, the greater the social desirability there is in a self-report measure to say 'yes, I do it' the harder it is to get accurate responses in a questionnaire, though there are ways to minimize this tendency, as discussed in Chapter 7.

Strangely enough though, if you ask people to record their own behaviour as it happens over a period of time, in a diary or log book, you can get reasonably accurate replies. Diary techniques have been shown useful in measuring people's diets, alcohol intake, number of cigarettes smoked per day and use of asthma medications.[7] Diaries do have some limitations however. Rather than simply being a method to record behaviour the diary can influence behaviour. For example, psychologists have known for some time that having clients write down every time they eat a piece of chocolate cake significantly modifies the client's intake. So in this case the diary is perhaps more a part of the intervention than of the evaluation. You will find that success with diary methods varies according to the format adopted, the extent to which they are checked by programme staff and the period of time within which they are used.[7] They are particularly useful, however, in recording behaviours or conditions that a person in your survey might not ordinarily recall with a high degree of accuracy if you were simply to try to ask them to give you an answer in an interview or one-off self-completed questionnaire. Such behaviours or conditions might include frequency of headaches, frequency of bed-wetting and the number of times a day a parent finds he or she loses their temper with their child.

How else can you measure behaviour? You can observe behaviour first hand. It may be inconvenient, but it may be the best choice in some circumstances. So you could observe, for example, the number of children who do and do not use the pedestrian crossing after school. You could observe the food choices people make at a factory canteen.

Sometimes you may not be able to do the observation yourself but you can do the next best thing. In trying to assess the food intake in a study which includes Greek and Italian migrants, for example, a team of researchers at Monash University in Melbourne have devised a simple method whereby people photograph what is on their plate before they eat it. A specially designed placemat with a geometric grid pattern on which the plate is placed is then used to estimate the food proportions.[8] But there may still be occasions where even your camera would not be welcome. Take for example occasions when you want to assess condom use! You may have to be satisfied with an indirect method of assessment, such as condom sales, though in Chapter 10 you will find a reference to some success in assessing condom use with a self-completed questionnaire.

Measuring health status

'Health' has a myriad of definitions. The appropriateness of a health status measure depends on the dimensions of health it measures relative to the sorts of effects you hope to detect. It is of no value, for example, to use as your measure of health status the number of times people are admitted to hospital, if your programme is trying to bring about changes in how people feel about themselves and how happily they relate to others in their social network.

Activity
How would you define health?

Feedback
Even though health is the basis of our work, out profession, our philosophy, you may find that defining it is not easy. The World Health Organization defines health as 'complete physical, mental and social

well being, and not merely the absence of infirmity'. Other definitions of health define it as those conditions which permit individuals to achieve their optimum capacity or realize their full potential. Health has positive or 'wellness' aspects, as well as disease or negative aspects.

Whatever definition you prefer, and there are many, you will find that there are dimensions within the concept of health that you may have to address more specifically as soon as you set out to measure health. A range of health status measures has been developed. Many of these are self-administered questionnaires which cover a variety of aspects such as physical abilities, for example the ability to care and manage for oneself, social interaction, social participation and contribution, anxiety, depression, self-control, family and work roles and illness events. Some measures focus on self-perception and self-assessment of health, such as asking people to rate their health on a scale from 'excellent' to 'poor'.

To choose a health status measure for your impact or outcome evaluation you must first clarify what the intended effect of the programme is likely to be and then choose a measure that taps the appropriate dimensions and a measure that is known to be suited to your target group. There are, for example, a whole range of health measures designed specifically for use with the elderly.[9] You should refer to Chapter 10 for an introduction to some measures that have been developed for measuring health status.

Measuring social support

There is an increasing body of evidence which indicates that people's social ties and social relationships affect their health. While the precise mechanisms for this remain unclear and research is proceeding (such as in the stress buffering role of social support), many health and community workers already have set up interventions to try to increase the quantity and quality of social support given to special target groups such as new parents, the recently bereaved, patients suffering from their first heart attack, newly arrived migrants and so on.

A range of self-completed questionnaires and interview schedules has been developed to measure social support. Some have been designed specifically for special target groups such as pregnant adolescents[10] and the elderly.[11]

Similarly to when you are selecting a health status measure, your selection of a measure for social support will depend on the emphasis you wish to place on the various dimensions of social support. These include, for example, the extent to which the social support network provides information, practical assistance, affirmation of personal worth and someone to lean on in times of crisis. Some measures focus on reciprocity within the network, that is, the extent to which help is received and given. Some measures focus on how well the network meets the individual's expectations or desired level of support. Your choice depends on what your programme is trying to achieve and what types of changes in the social support network you consider to be important. Chapter 10 may assist you in locating some of these measures.

Remember too that your investigation of the effects of social support could simply be largely unstructured and qualitative. If you are running, for example, a fairly simple programme to link up isolated families in a new housing estate, it may be quite inappropriate to get them to fill out lengthy questionnaires when it comes to measuring your programme's impact on social support. Some of the dimensions covered in these instruments, however, could guide your approach or line of questioning.

One simple and easy measure of young families' social network which has been frequently used is recording the names of children invited to attend each other's birthday parties. Another measure is to find out, for example, how many women in your discussion group can give you the names of each other's spouses and children or can tell you that they have visited each other's homes or telephoned each other since first meeting each other at your programme.

Measuring quality of life

In times past, many programmes were evaluated in terms of the length of time or years the programme added to life. Now, the saying goes that the emphasis should also be to 'add life to years'. In other words, in evaluating health promotion and disease prevention programmes, the emphasis should be on making life rewarding, enjoyable and productive and not simply long.

Again, as with measurement of social support, your approach to assessing the impact of your programme on quality of life could be simple, unstructured and open; you could go to your participants and ask them 'Has the programme improved the way you live your life? Your enjoyment? The range of things you can now do and share with other people?' and so on. On the other hand you could take advantage of the range of self-completed questionnaires and interview schedules that has been developed specifically to measure quality of life. These have been developed for the general population[12] and for particular target groups, such as cancer patients.[13]

The sorts of dimensions covered by these instruments are similar to some of the health status measures. They include the capacity of the individual to function independently (to take care of themselves without help from others), the extent to which they feel anxious or depressed, the extent to which they feel they are making a useful contribution (to work, to family or to society), how well they feel and so on. Chapter 10 indicates where you might locate some of these measures.

Measuring costs

The price of something is not the same as its cost and neither may be equivalent to its worth or value.

When you are running a programme, what will be the marginal cost of adding additional participants? What are the capital costs compared to the cost of disposables? What is the opportunity cost of the programme? That is, by allocating resources to one programme, what does this mean in terms of programmes we have now lost the opportunity to run? When you measure costs, should you cost over one session? One set of sessions? One year?

These are just some of the things that have to be considered before you can start to assess programme costs or health costs. It is likely that administrators will want some information on programme costs, but costing is also a difficult thing to do well and different people will argue about which might be the best way to measure costs. If you are being encouraged to look at costs, and we suggest you do so, particularly after you have first established programme effectiveness, we suggest that you contact a health economist for some advice. Chapter 11 on consultants will provide some guidance about this.

Measuring community strength, 'competence' or participation

In the evaluation of community development programmes, it has been argued that programme success cannot be adequately assessed by health measures taken on individuals within that community. This would not adequately capture the nature of the community development outcomes. Success is linked with changes in the community itself, its networks, its structures, the way in which people perceive the community, ownership of community issues, perceived and actual 'empowerment' in health and social issues. A community that undergoes community development presumably changes in relation to these sorts of factors. While qualitative case examples may capture people's accounts of these changes, measurement of these changes in the quantitative sense is also progressing.

As with measurement of many of the factors that have been discussed up to this point, measurement of community level factors first requires conceptual clarification of the sorts of effects that the intervention is likely to bring about and the sorts of changes within dimensions of the community that you would hope to detect with your evaluation. This should lead back to your intentions and reaffirmation of the model or philosophy of your approach. In other words, as mentioned right at the beginning, evaluation depends on values. For example, do you want your community groups to have success in attracting resources to the community or is it sufficient for them simply to develop the skills that could bring about this eventuality? Is the success of the intervention determined just by whether the community

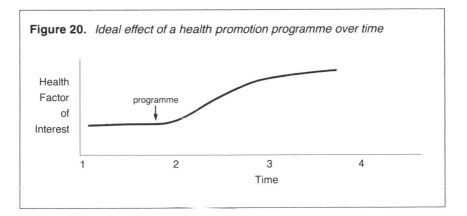

Figure 20. *Ideal effect of a health promotion programme over time*

'feels good' about it, or is there a risk that you could allow a community to become satisfied, unjustifiably? Has the intervention made a difference to community problem solving capacity?

Systematic measurement approaches in this field are still developing. Some researchers have developed measures of community 'strength' or 'competence' that assess community functioning and capacity to deal with community concerns and these involve surveys of community members. Some of the dimensions covered by these scales include, for example, 'commitment' (how residents value the importance of the community), 'articulateness' (how well components of the community are able to express their views), 'participation' (active contribution towards the definition and achievement of community goals), 'conflict containment and accommodation' (effective recognition and management of differences).[14] In other areas the instrument development is lagging as people still struggle with identifying the dimensions of interest, such as the dimensions which indicate the nature and stages of community empowerment from awareness of a problem to caring about a problem and then making a commitment to change it.[15]

This is an exciting and promising new area and these developments encourage health workers to think about what they are trying to achieve. Remember not to let yourself end up equating effort with success or let 'participation' mask the need for some agreement about what all parties might consider satisfactory achievements or endpoints. Agreement on this might indeed be part of the 'vision' and intervention itself.

When are Effects Likely to Occur?

When do you think your programme is going to demonstrate its effects? The day after it ends? One week later? One month later? Three months later? This is very important because you don't want to make

116 EVALUATING HEALTH PROMOTION

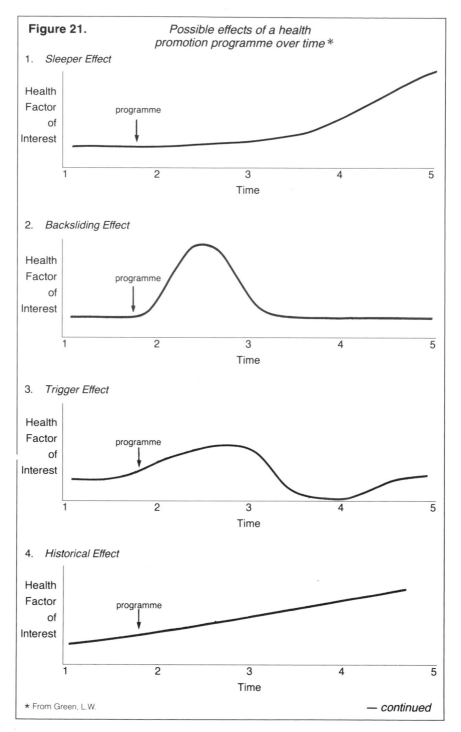

Figure 21. *Possible effects of a health promotion programme over time**

1. *Sleeper Effect*
2. *Backsliding Effect*
3. *Trigger Effect*
4. *Historical Effect*

* From Green, L.W. — *continued*

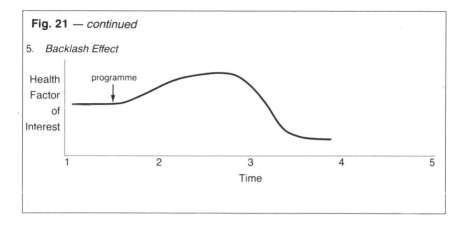

Fig. 21 — *continued*

5. *Backlash Effect*

a mistake of choosing a time to measure your effects when its too early or too late.

The ideal effect of a health promotion programme is illustrated in Figure 20. In this illustration we see that the impact of the programme has been an immediate improvement in the health factor of interest and this is sustained over time.

Unfortunately, in the real world, health promotion rarely has instantaneous and everlasting effects. However, effects may still be sufficient to be worthwhile. A leading authority in health promotion evaluation, Lawrence Green, has suggested that the real effects of programmes may fall into five different categories as illustrated in Figure 21.[16]

With the sleeper effect, the impact of a programme delivered at T2 (time 2) would be undetected if the health worker measured effects only at T3 (time 3). The effect, as it turns out, is only apparent at T4 and T5.

With the backsliding effect, on the other hand, the effect is immediate but short lasting. If a health worker made only a single measurement at T4 or T5, the programme's effect would be missed. This can happen with some behaviour modification programmes, such as weight control, where without the discipline of the weekly sessions and regimen participants can fall quickly back into old habits.

The trigger effect has also been called 'borrowing from the future' because it triggers or brings forward a behaviour or event that would have happened anyway. An example might be a Pap smear campaign that may show an increase in the number of women presenting for Pap smears in August (which looks like a success or big improvement) when in fact these women would have ordinarily presented for a Pap smear in September or October. Immediately after the programme an effect is apparent (T3) but by T4 the level has dropped down even lower than before the programme. At T5 the level has returned to normal.

The historical effect illustrates the fact that in many cases a health behaviour or factor may be gradually improving across time: your evaluation may 'capture' this effect and wrongly attribute it to the programme. These secular trends (such as increases in consumption of low-fat foods, decreases in heart disease mortality) need to be distinguished from programme effects. Evaluation designs that may help to do this are discussed in the next section.

Backlash effects occur when premature cessation of the programme demoralizes or embitters participants, leading to levels of behaviours or problems that are worse than before the programme started. An example might be street kids' drug-taking and risk-taking behaviour after the close of a community refuge or withdrawal of a community education worker. Again, if measurement of effect only occurred at T2 the true impact of the programme and its subsequent effects would go unrecognized and misinterpreted.

How do you know which scenario is going to apply to your own situation? The answer is to consult the literature and see what other people have shown. You should also think out the problem carefully. For example, is yours the sort of programme where people might be careful in the one or two weeks after the programme ends but then lapse into old behaviour patterns? Alternatively, is yours the sort of programme where people really need to have a certain time period after the programme before the effect 'matures' or before people have had sufficient opportunity to practise the new skills they may have learned?

If you really have no idea what will happen you should conduct a small pilot study. Rather then taking all your participants and measuring them all at one point in time, which you are uncertain about, it would be better to take just a small group and take several measures over a period of time. In this way you may pick up when the effects occur and this will help you to plan your main study.

Evaluation Designs: How can you be Sure that your Programme Caused the Effects you Observe?

Activity

Let's say that a health surveyor sets up a reminder system to send out cards to parents to remind them that their child's vaccination is due. Because 90% of parents do present their children for vaccination at the clinic in the next two months, he concludes that his reminder programme is a success. Do you agree with his conclusion?

Consider another example. A student health officer conducts an extensive series of AIDS education programmes in tertiary colleges. At the end of the programme, 60% of students say that they would not have sex without a condom. She concludes that the programme is a success. Do you agree with her conclusion?

Finally, a psychologist conducts a series of stress management workshops for a large public service department. Two months after the end of the workshops her results show that stress levels and days off work are considerably less for the people who attended the workshops compared to a sample of those office workers who didn't come along. In her report to the Public Service Board she recommends that stress management workshops be set up across all government departments. Would you support this recommendation?

Feedback

Essentially, the main problem with each of these examples is that there may be other explanations as to why the 'effects' observed occured. In the case of the immunization reminder system, the real reason why 90% of parents had their children vaccinated might have been because the state government ran a media campaign about immunization at the same time. Unless we know how many students usually use condoms, we can't assess whether the AIDS education programme made any impact. Finally, the stress management workshops may have only attracted those office workers sensitive to their stress levels and willing and able to do something about it. So-called 'success' with this group may have been easy, but it may not have been so easy with those people who didn't volunteer to attend. Another explanation may be that those people who came along actually experience less stress than the people who did not attend.

All these problems can be addressed in the design of the evaluation study. A number of different types of designs have traditionally been used in evaluation research. The designs vary in quality (that is, in how good the evidence is that the design produces), complexity, and in the time and resources that go into their execution. A number of these designs will now be presented, with a short discussion on the value of each. The taxonomy for these designs is based on the work of Cook and Campbell.[17]

Single group, post-test only

Here you take measurement at the end of the programme only, and only on the people who were exposed to the programme (for example, your programme participants in a group-based education programme, or the viewing audience in a television-based campaign). Like with the immunization example given earlier, the problem with this design is that you can't be sure about two things. Firstly, did a change actually occur? Or were 90% of parents going to get their children vaccinated anyway? Secondly, can you be sure that it really was your reminder system and nothing else that caused what you have interpreted as an effect?

Single group, pre-test and post-test

Here you make two measurements, one before and one after the programme. The advantage of this design over the former one is that it is set up to detect change. However, you still can't be sure that something else is not causing the effects you see.

Non-equivalent control group, pre-test and post-test

In evaluation research when people talk about a control group or a comparison group they are referring to a group of people who don't receive your programme, but whose behaviour or conditions are monitored in order to compare them to the people who do receive your programme. If the people who don't receive your programme get worse or stay the same while the people who get your programme improve, then this provides evidence that your programme is working, that is, it can be concluded that your programme is causing the effects you observe.

In this design you have two groups, the experimental or programme group (the people who get the programme) and the control or comparison group. Measurements are made on both groups before and after the programme in order to detect change in the factor of interest. That is, does it get better, get worse or stay the same?

The words 'non-equivalent' to describe your control group refer to the fact that the people in your experimental group and the people in your control group do not share the exact same characteristics. This may happen when you draw your control group from another municipality, or from another state, or another hospital ward. Maybe the control group came from another time period, like when you are comparing the effects of your patient education programme run in March, April and May with a control group of patients that were admitted to hospital in June, July and August. There are ways to effectively choose an 'equivalent' control group and these are discussed later.

The before and after aspect of this design gives it strength. However, the fact that your two groups are considered 'non-equivalent' can be a concern. This is because if these two groups differ in some way it may be that it is these differences and not the effect of your programme that account for the before and after changes you might see in the groups. For example, it may be that your programme works because the people in your programme group are better educated than the people in your control group. Maybe they are fitter, or generally more active.

For differences between your two groups that you know about, such as age or asthma severity, it is possible to analyse your data in a particular way to adjust for these differences and thereby exclude their influence. When you can do this it makes the evaluation design much stronger. There may still be a worry though about the differences

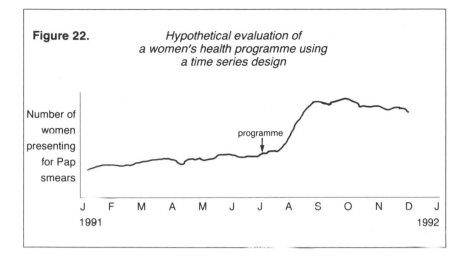

Figure 22. Hypothetical evaluation of a women's health programme using a time series design

between the groups which are unknown to you and which may bias your results and interpretation.

Single group, time series
Sometimes the problem of teasing out programme effects from those differences arising because of non-equivalent groups is so difficult that people opt to simply do more before and after measures on the programme group. It may also be that it is impossible to find a suitable control group.

Lots of measures over a period of time is called a time series. In this way you are able to observe natural changes occuring in the group and the size and direction of these changes before you introduce your intervention and observe its effect.

In the example in Figure 22, you can see how attendances for Pap smears at women's health centres across the state were gradually increasing from January to July. In August a large increase in attendances was recorded, coinciding with a media-promoted women's health education programme. In the months after the campaign the levels of attendances dropped slightly but remained above pre-campaign levels, indicating perhaps increased awareness in the community.

This provides pretty strong evidence for the programme having caused the effect observed. This is because of the opportunity to observe a long period before and after the programme. The only rival explanation would be that some phenomenon occurred in exactly the same time period, and it would be usual to try to consider what this might be and discount it if appropriate.

Non-equivalent groups, time series

This design is a combination of the two above and it provides even stronger evidence for concluding that the programme really caused the effects observed. This is because it more definitely rules out rival explanations as to why the effects occurred by introducing the control group again. The design is also better than design 3 (non-equivalent groups with a pre-test and a post-test) because serial measurements on both groups well before and well after the intervention help to cancel out secular trends or historical effects. That is, they give a good indication of what is happening with your population over time before you examine the independent effects of your programme.

An example of this design would be the evaluation of your Pap smear campaign, as discussed above, where you included data on Pap smears in other states across the same time period. You would ensure that the states chosen had no campaigns of this nature running at the same time.

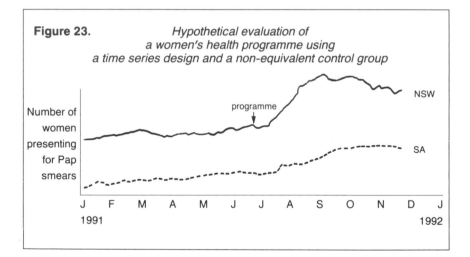

Figure 23. *Hypothetical evaluation of a women's health programme using a time series design and a non-equivalent control group*

Randomized controlled trial

The final design which overcomes all of the problems of the designs listed before is the randomized controlled trial. In the terminology we have been using, the longer name for this design would be 'equivalent groups, pre-test and post-test' or if more measures were taken before and after 'equivalent groups, time series'. If this design is so good, why don't we just run these all the time and dispense with the other designs? Because it is not always possible to conduct randomized controlled trials. Mostly, this is due to the sort of control group in these trials.

Up until now we have been using the words 'control group' and 'comparison group' interchangeably, as most people do. However, strictly speaking, the words 'control group' should only refer to a group which can be considered to be alike in every way to the experimental or programme group, except for the fact that they were not exposed to your programme. According to statistical theory, the only way in which you can be sure of this is if people are allocated to the control group or the experimental group entirely by chance. The only time this can happen is when you are doing random allocation (flipping a coin or using a random number table).

You can see that with random allocation, with both groups being alike in every way, it can be inferred that any difference you observe between your groups after the programme must have been caused by your programme. A randomized controlled trial is considered to be a true experiment. All the other designs presented up to this point are called 'quasi-experimental'.

Under what sorts of circumstances can you randomly allocate people to experimental or control groups? Let's take a group-based smoking cessation programme. A health educator advertises in the local newspaper that a stop smoking group will commence shortly at the local community health centre. The ideal group size is say 10 people per group. Twenty-five people telephone the centre in the next week and ask to be enrolled in the programme. How would you determine who got into the programme first and who had to wait for the next one? You could allocate on a first-come first-served basis. However, this might mean that all your people in your experimental group could be considered more keen to stop smoking because they telephoned first. For them, success may come more easily than for the people on your waiting list (who could become your control group) because people on the waiting list might be a little different. This is the ideal circumstance where you could randomly allocate people to groups with little difficulty.

When is it hard to get an equivalent control group? The most obvious answer to this is when your intervention is so broad that it is hard to prevent people from being exposed to it, such as with media approaches or community development approaches. In these circumstances the only possible control group would be people living in another state or region, who although they may have some similar characteristics, would have to be considered non-equivalent. People have, however, been quite inventive when it comes to random allocation. If you can't randomly allocate individuals to your programme, you can instead randomly allocate other units, such as classrooms of school children or schools or neighbourhoods. This means that the data analysis has to be conducted a little differently, but it means that the study retains the strength of a randomized design.

What Evaluation Design should a Fieldworker Choose?

The implication from the section above on evaluation designs is that some designs are better than others, in that they produce stonger evidence about programme effects, but some designs are easier to execute than others so a balance needs to be reached.

What evaluation design should a fieldworker choose? The reason for raising this question is because the opportunities that the people who deliver programmes have for research are limited. Many of the designs we have listed require data to be collected from programme participants or from the target group on many occasions when you would not ordinarily see these people for your programme. That is, for example, when serial measurements are taken on factors over a long period of time. The situation is also true when you consider that including a control group in your evaluation design may mean that you take measures from a group of people whom you may not ordinarily come into contact with, such as people in neighbouring regions or populations in other states.

These considerations lead to the conclusion that the people who design and run health promotion programmes are unlikely to have the opportunity to also become personally involved in long time series designs or designs that involve control groups. When a programme requires this sort of evaluation, more evaluation resources will be required. You may need the assistance of a research officer to collect experimental and control groups and make measures. Should your evaluation require a very large sample size (see Chapters 7 and 11) you may need to have several people collecting data. It is not unusual for the evaluation budget for these types of studies to range from $10 000 to over $100 000 for very large community field trials.

When is this sort of input going to be justified? From your process evaluation and your evaluability assessment you can see that you would only want evaluation of this scale to proceed when the programme is likely to work, if it is ever going to work. That is, when the programme is well implemented and you are satisfied with programme reach and quality. But what about some indication of programme effects? You want to make sure that you will avoid misinterpreting programme effects, such as when you may have sleeper effects and so on. You may also want to be assured that some type of effect is there before you start spending your evaluation resources on taking measurements in a control group.

A practical and feasible solution to this problem is for the fieldworker to undertake some preliminary asessment of programme effects, using a single group, pre-test and post-test design, before a decision is made to mount resources to launch a more complicated evaluation design. That way, if you detect no effect at all, you can find out why and reconsider your intervention before it is subjected to more rigorous evaluation.

We therefore suggest that this is the way you should proceed. The person responsible for the programme can select the appropriate way to measure the factor of interest (possibly after some consultation) and proceed to use the measure before and after the programme with a group of, say, 40 or so people. With this size group you should be able to analyse the data needing not much more than a pocket calculator. If there is no inkling of an effect you should go back and see why and improve your programme accordingly. If there is an effect then one of the 'higher order' designs can be launched to see if you can really attribute this effect to your programme.

A note of caution. You may be familiar with a concept known as 'statistical significance'. It refers to the probability that you would have observed an effect similar to the one you did observe just by chance, even if there were no real effect at all. When someone says that the effect was statistically significant, for example, when they say that there was a significant increase in the proportion of children immunized in an area before and after a programme, what they usually mean is that the probability of this increase occurring 'by accident' is less than 5%. Because the chance is so low, you can say that it is reasonable to conclude that the programme worked.

Unfortunately, when you are using just small sample sizes, you may not be able to pick up a statistically significant and important effect even if it is there. That is, if your group was larger, a reduction you might have shown in smoking may be statistically significant, but because you have only a small group, the size of effect you might consider important may not be detected. What happens then? Won't you risk making the wrong conclusions about your programme?

Before we answer that question let's consider another scenario. Let's suppose that the way in which you have chosen to measure your factor of interest has biassed your results. Let's say that the way you chose to measure people's correct use of medications was self-report. Maybe the reason it looks like your medication education programme is successful is because people simply told you they were taking their medications properly at the end, regardless of the truth. Here your programme will be showing an effect when in fact there may not be a true effect. Your choice of measuring instrument is very important, and measurement issues have been discussed in this chapter. Chapter 10 will help you choose a measuring instrument in health promotion and Chapter 11 talks about the sort of people that may also be able to advise you.

However, after you have completed a single group pre-test post-test design, it is still possible that the effect you have observed has been exaggerated by your measuring instruments or disguised by your sample size. There also may be circumstances where your measure masks a true effect. These problems can only be sorted out with further help and resources.

For example, it may be necessary to 'validate' your self-report questionnaire for measuring drug compliance by comparing the results you get from it with a better measure of drug compliance, say physiological markers in people's urine. If you get similar answers from both, you can say that your questionnaire is a valid measure and you can use it with confidence. If the results from using the two approaches are very different, you can't use your questionnaire; it is not a valid measure. That is, it is not a good measure of what it purports to measure. Further, it may be necessary to double or treble your sample size in order to be able to detect an important and statistically significant result.

Validation studies of measuring instruments are separate pieces of research within themselves. They require special skills in research design and data analysis. They can take many months. Increasing your sample size, as we have mentioned, will always entail securing additional resources. Either way, the people who can help you, researchers, evaluators, epidemiologists and so on, will need the data from you preliminary study to help them plan the next stages. Data from your preliminary study including your qualitative investigation of programme effects, should also provide sufficient justification that the effect you may have demonstrated is worth pursuing.

Why is impact and outcome evaluation worth all this trouble? Because when we argue for more resources for health promotion programmes we want to be sure that the evidence we provide about the effectiveness of these interventions cannot be faulted. At the very least, the evidence for health promotion effectiveness should be as good as the evidence put forward for justifying competing expenditures elsewhere in the health care system, such as the evaluative trials put forward to justify high-technology treatment units.

The important thing to remember is that to do your programme justice, the evaluation and the evaluation resources devoted to it should be adequate. This means that you must be clear about what you can and cannot do within the programme resources and you must seek additional funding for evaluation research as necessary. Funding authorities commonly expect more in the evaluations of programmes than they match in funds allocated and it is up to you to educate them about what is and what is not possible. It is far better to have the results from a well-executed process evaluation than to produce data from a poor and prematurely conducted randomized controlled trial. Here we may have the situation of a potentially good programme being buried as the result of a bad evaluation. Fortunately, some funding authorities are getting this message.

Results from your preliminary studies should form the basis of your submission for additional evaluation funds. You must then work closely and effectively with the additional people that may come on the scene (researchers, statisticians and so on) to make sure that the essence of your programme, and what it is trying to achieve, are appropriately addressed. No amount of additional research skill and technology can replace the contribution of the programme staff and originators.

References

1. Green, LW. Should health education abandon attitude change strategies? Perspectives from recent research. *Health Education Monographs* 1970;30:25–48.

2. Scriven M. The pros and cons of goal free evaluation. *Evaluation Comment* 1972;3(4):1–7.

3. Dwyer T, Pierce JP, Hannam CD, Burke N. Evaluation of the Sydney 'Quit for Life. Campaign' Part 2 Changes in smoking prevalence. *Medical Journal of Australia* 1986;144:33–347.

4. Hill DJ, Gray NJ. Patterns of tobacco smoking in Australia. *Medical Journal of Australia* 1982;1:23–25.

5. Webb GR, Bowman J, Sanson-Fisher R. Studies of Child safety restraints in motor vehicles: some methodological considerations. *Accident Analysis and Prevention* 1988;20:109–115.

6. Hawe P, Wilson A, Fahey P, Field P, Cunningham AJ, Baker M, Leeder SR The validity of parental report as a measure of a child's measles immunisation status. Submitted for publication.

7. Verbrugge LM. Health diaries. *Medical Care* 1980;13(1):73–95.

8. Powles J, Ktenas D, Sutherland C, Hage B. Food habits in Southern European migrants: a case study of migrants from the Greek island of Levkada. In: Truswell AS, Walquist ML (eds). *Food Habits in Australia*. Melbourne: Rene Gordon, 1988.

9. Kane RA, Kane RL. *Assessing the Elderly. A Practical Guide to Measurement.* Lexington, Massachusetts: Lexington Books, 1981.

10. Barrera M. Social support in the adjustment of pregnant adolescents: assessment issues. In: Gottlieb BII (ed) *Social Networks and Social Support* Beverly Hills: Sage, 1981;69–96.

11. Henderson AS, Grayson DA, Scott R, Wilson J, Rickwood D, Kay DWK. Social support, dementia and depression among the elderly living in the Hobart community. *Psychological Medicine* 1986;16:379–390.

12. Kind P. *The Design and Construction of Quality of Life Measures*. Discussion Paper 43. Centre for Health Economics University of York, Heslington, York.

13. Spitzer WO, Dobson AJ, Hall J, Chesterman E, Levi J, Shepherd R, Battista RN, Cathlove BR. Measuring quality of life in cancer patients. A concise QL index for use by physicians. *Journal of Chronic Diseases* 1981;34(12):585–597.

14. Goeppinger J, Baglioni AJ. Community competence: a positive approach to needs assessment. *American Journal of Community Psychology* 1985;13(5): 507–523.

15. Swift C, Levin G. Empowerment: an emerging mental health technology. *Journal of Primary Prevention* 1987;8(1,2)71–94.

16. Green, LW. Evaluation and measurement: some dilemmas for health education *American Journal of Public Health* 1977;67:155–161.

17. Cook TD, Campbell DT. *Quasi-experimentation. Design and Analysis Issues for Field Settings*. Chicago: Rand McNally Publishing, 1979.

Further Reading

Braverman MT. (ed.) *Evaluating Promotion Programs. New Directions for Program Evaluation*, No. 43. San Francisco: Jossey Bass, Fall 1989

PART 2

Programme Evaluation: The Skills You Need

Chapter 7

SURVEY METHODS
AND QUESTIONNAIRE DESIGN

OBJECTIVES

At the end of this chapter you should be able to:

1. Specify a survey question.
2. List different types of sampling techniques and their advantages and disadvantages.
3. Calculate the amount of time and resources you would need for your survey.
4. Identify the main types of question formats and the occasions appropriate to their use.
5. List the main modes of data collection and their advantages and disadvantages.
6. Analyse the results of your survey and put these into a written report.

In needs assessment and in evaluation there will be occasions when you may need to collect large amounts of information from lots of people or from lots of documents or records. To collect this data both efficiently and accurately you will need to rely on good survey design and good questionnaire design. In the last few decades there has been an explosion in survey research and researchers have taken the opportunity to study how to sample populations and how to word questions so that they get accurate and reliable information, with least cost. Survey techniques have improved over time and recommendations from field research in this area have been put into a variety of articles and texts, some of which are listed at the end of this chapter. Here we will condense some of this wisdom and alert you to the main considerations in planning your survey and designing your questionnaire.

Ingredients of a Survey

The survey consists of a number of components and we will be considering each of these in turn.

The survey questions	*what you want to know*
The sample	*who to recruit for your survey and how you will find them*
Survey planning	*mode of inquiry, timing, resource considerations, cost*
The questionnaire	*the survey instrument, content and wording of questions, formats for answers, question sequence*
Response rates	*respondents' cooperation with your survey, response bias*
The analysis	*making sense of qualitative and quantitative data*
The report	*putting it all into an attractive and easy-to-understand form*

Survey Questions

Activity

Consider the following question that staff at a cardiac rehabilitation unit have set out to investigate: Are people attending the programme satisfied with the quality of care they receive?' What would you need to do before you could set out to conduct a survey to answer this question?

Feedback

This question gives you the general idea of what staff want to know but it is impossible to investigate it just yet because it is too vague. What people are they referring to? All people that have ever attended the unit or just those in the last six months? What do they mean by 'quality of care'? Do they mean waiting times? Appointment times? Sensitivity of the staff? Friendliness of ward staff? How welcome their families are made to feel? How well staff answer their questions and give further information?

The question should also be made more specific in another way. Look at the way it is presently phrased: 'Are people satisfied . . . ?' Chances are that the answer to this question is not going to be 'yes' or 'no'. Some people will be satisfied and others will not be. It would be far better to phrase the question: 'What proportion of people are satisfied . . . ?' This way the real extent of feeling on the issue could be assessed.

This should illustrate that before you can set out to answer a survey question you must first ensure that it is stated very specifically. You need to state exactly who your question refers to, the dimensions of the variables you are interested in and the time frame you intend to operate within. You can see that this is a bit akin to specifying a programme goal or objective by time, person, place and amount. A good way to think about it is to try to state your question so specifically that a person other than yourself could set out to answer it in a manner you consider appropriate.

There are reasons for being at pains to be clear about this at the outset. Firstly, clear questions at the beginning will take a lot of the frustration out of the later questionnaire design (that is, you will be free to concentrate on design issues with question formats and not content issues). Secondly, if you take care with this step and all parties agree, you will avoid the unhappy but common scenario of getting to the end of the analysis of your results and finding that your survey missed the collection of some vital information.

The Sample

From whom are you going to collect information? In most cases you will be collecting data from people, but often the subjects of your survey will be medical records or documents of some kind. In either case you still have to face the likely situation that you may not always be able to survey everybody connected with your field of interest (because of the sheer size of this group) and you will be forced to take a sample and try to infer from them what the result would be if you really were able to survey everybody.

Types of samples

The best sort of sample is what is known as a *random sample*. It works like this. Let's say that 200 people have attended your weight loss courses and you want to interview 50 of them to find out how they have been managing since they completed the programme. With random selection of these subjects each person has the same chance as each other person to be selected into your group. In other words the selection is fair and there is no bias in favour of choosing some people over others. The sample chosen using this method is considered to be representative.

To choose a random sample you can use a random number table from the back of an elementary statistics text. First of all you have to number all your people from 1 to 200. You then read from the table which people to select from this group (for example, 006, 023, 056, 078, 189, 034 . . .) and you continue to do so until you have collected your 50 people. Just ignore numbers larger than 200 in the table.

Let's consider another situation. Let's say that you want to survey 50 people enrolling for weight control courses in your area for interviews to find out what previous methods they have used to lose weight. There would be a method to take a random sample of these people but the problem you may have is that the student you have working with you to conduct the interviews only works with you on Wednesday afternoons. It may be that although people call up to enrol in classes each day of the week your sample can only consist of people selected because they called in on a Wednesday afternoon. This is called *systematic sampling*. Another common method of systematic sampling is to take every third person on a list or every tenth caller to a hotline. The advantage of systematic sampling when you are accruing subjects prospectively is that it is predicatable. That is, you know when you need to be prepared to collect data. However, systematic sampling may produce some bias in your results if there is something peculiar about the method for identifying subjects that you have chosen. For example, many people consider that the GP patients lined up on a Monday morning are a biased group compared to the people who visit GPs later in the week. So systematically taking patients into a study from Monday morning only may give you a picture quite different from that which might have been obtained if you had taken a sample of patients from every day of the week.

Another type of sample is the *convenience sample*. Quite simply, these are people who you can get to easily. For example, they might be people you approach to answer questions in a shopping centre or people who you ask to fill out your questionnaire at a display you might have set up at a health fair. Like the systematic sample, this method of sampling illustrates how your methods are often constrained by your resources and opportunities. Again, the type of people you 'capture' by this method may not reflect the whole group about which you wish to make inferences. Frequently people using this method of sampling ask their respondents questions about their sociodemographic characteristics, so that they can at least directly determine whether their sample was younger than the area's population as a whole, better educated and so on. This gives an indication of the nature of the bias you might have in your sample because of the method you chose to select your sample.

The final method of sampling that is sometimes used is called *snowball sampling*. This is where you locate subjects for your survey by asking your existing subjects to nominate someone for you from their own network. It is frequently used in surveys of hard-to-get-to populations such as intravenous drug users, homosexuals, homeless youth and recently arrived migrant groups. Critics of this method are concerned that the people recruited by this method represent a biased group. That is, the network of people recruited by this method would not have the same characteristics as a sample of the same sort of people chosen by random selection. However, the point of this approach is that you can't select the sample by alternative means. Proponents of snowball sampling argue that without it you would have no way to identify a sample at all and therefore no data to provide a basis for needs assessment and programme development. Some data, they argue, is better than none at all.

Sample size

How big should your sample be? This depends on how precise you want your results to be. Another consideration is how much data you can afford to collect and how vital this particular survey is in the overall programme development and evaluation plan you may have. This is an important point and worth a moment to illustrate.

First of all you must remember that when you take a sample from a population and study it, you are not simply interested in the people in your sample. What you are really trying to do is to use the sample to say something about the population which you feel they represent. So if you take a sample of new mothers attending postnatal clinics and interview them, your intention may be to design a programme for all new mothers in your area and not just for the women you interviewed. If you measure cholesterol levels at a health fair, you want to use the information to make general statements about the problem of high cholesterol in your community. Statisticians are interested in the statistical theory of probability that provides an estimate of how likely it is that the result you obtained from your sample is the same as that for the whole population. You are hardly ever going to be exactly right so what can be calculated instead is the range of values within which we can say the true value in the population is likely to lie.

Generally speaking, the bigger your sample the more precise your estimate or result is likely to be. Let's say, for example, that you have done a survey of forty 13 and 14 year old high school students and found that 16 of them (40%) admit to drinking alcohol at least once a week. If you then went to see a statistician he or she could tell you that you could only conclude from this that the true proportion of children in your population that are regular drinkers is actually likely to range anywhere between 25% and 57% (using a statistical concept known as 'confidence intervals').

Let's say that you decide that this range of values is far too wide and you want to get a more precise estimate of the problem before you set out to design an intervention. Now that you have an idea that the size of the problem could be in the order of 40%, your statistician can advise you what sample size you would need to get a precise estimate (that is, an estimate within a range of values that is not too wide). So with a sample size of 90 children, for example, and a result from your survey that 40% are regular drinkers you could conclude that the true proportion in the population is likely to be within the range of 30% to 51%. With a sample size of 400 (and a result from your survey of 40%) the range of values within which the true population value almost certainly lies is 35% to 45%. So you have to get into large numbers before your estimates start becoming quite precise.

Do you always need to go to the trouble of collecting precise estimates? This depends on the purpose of your survey. If you are setting up a needs assessment to determine the sorts of problems in the community and the factors contributing to these problems in order to design an intervention, it could be argued that the precision of your estimates is not as important as the actual nature of the data you collect and how well it illustrates the dynamics of the problem. In other words, it may be more important for your data to tell you why children are drinking, where they drink, when they drink, with whom and so on, than it is to get the exact proportion who are regular drinkers very precisely. On the other hand, if your data are also going to be used as the 'pre' measure or baseline measure against which you will be evaluating the success of your intervention, then your estimate of the proportion who drink regularly will need to be fairly precise as otherwise you will have difficulty detecting the effect of your intervention when you compare your 'pre' and 'post' assessments.

What about the resource implications of sample size in surveys? In the next section we concentrate on what you can usefully do with limited resources. Again, it should be stressed that if at any time in the process of the research activities you carry out for needs assessment or for evaluation you decide that what is really required is something bigger than what you can accomplish yourself, then you should devote your energies to submitting for more resources. This is preferable to having the development of the programme limited by the research activity a single person can achieve on their own. You should remember, however, that your own work is critically important and lays the foundation for what may be taken up by others subsequently. For example, no statistician can give advice about the sample size needed for a survey without someone being able to first give him or her an estimate of the size of the problem under investigation. In other words, in the example above, without someone having first surveyed the drinking habits of 40 schoolchildren to ascertain that 40% were regular drinkers, none of the subsequent planning for larger scale surveys could have taken place.

Survey Planning

Mode of inquiry

Your first consideration should be how you are going to collect your data. The most common methods are *face-to-face interviews, telephone surveys* and *self-completed questionnaires* which can be mailed to respondents. The method you choose will depend on the sort of data you wish to collect. For example, if you are just after descriptive information such as the size of the family, children's ages and what childcare services the family uses, then this sort of data could easily be filled out by subjects in a questionnaire. However, if your project is more exploratory and you want to find out people's broad views or attitudes (like what they think are the needs of young families in the area, or their negative and positive experiences in using services) you might be better collecting this data in an interview (face to face or over the phone). This is because people may have a lot to say, a lot you could not anticipate, and you would also tire respondents if you expected them to write it all down for you. So, in the first instance, your choice about your mode of inquiry will rest on whether you are attempting to collect largely qualitative data or quantitative data.

Another thing that governs the choice of mode of inquiry is the extent to which you feel able to structure the line of questioning you wish to pursue. With a *structured approach* you set a line of questioning in your survey and all respondents are led through it. The inflexibility thus limits the opportunity for the respondent to add information which they feel is important or related. On the other hand, the approach does guarantee that all respondents consider the same issues or topics so their results can be compared with each other and easily summarized.

With an *unstructured approach* the person being interviewed is allowed to take the lead and talk about whatever aspects of the survey topic he or she chooses. The strength of this approach is that it often reveals issues and ideas that you, the survey designer, might have never considered. The respondent's view and opinion is unique. This is the essence of the qualitative approach. However, because respondents are not systematically led through certain question areas, you may be left uncertain about the way all respondents feel about some issues.

The unstructured approach can only really be undertaken successfully in a face-to-face interview or in a focus group as it is hard to establish the rapport needed for this to work well in other situations.

Structured approaches can suit any mode, but even in self-completed questionnaires most researchers leave scope for respondents to add their own ideas and comments that may have come to mind as a result of the questions. So it is possible to combine the best of the two approaches.

Very commonly researchers may start out researching a topic using unstructured face-to-face interviews and then as time goes on, and as they become familiar with the range of responses and ideas that people come up with, their survey method may move more towards structured approaches. So, after a few initial rounds of qualitative interviews with relatively small samples to build up a picture of the sorts of dimensions of a problem or issue, a researcher may start to construct questions which could form the basis of later quantitative investigations of the same problem using self-completed questionnaires with larger groups of people. Indeed this is the usual way in which people develop measures for a wide range of psychological, attitudinal, health and social factors. Barrera, for example, has built on this approach in the development of his instrument to measure social support received by pregnant adolescents.[1]

Many researchers undertake surveys incorporating both modes of investigation. Table 12 compares face-to-face interviews, telephone interviews and mailed self-completed questionnaires on a number of parameters. Later discussion will return to some of these issues.

Resources and timing

Keeping in mind that your principal role is programme provider and not researcher, how much time should you devote to your survey and how much should you expect to accomplish in that time? First of all as a general rule it takes as long to analyse data as it does to collect it. Add to this the time you spend in survey planning and in writing up a report. Let's suppose that the survey forms the main basis of your needs assessment or impact or outcome evaluation. We would advise that you spend no more than one month collecting data. Add to this one month of planning, preparation and pilot testing, one month for analysis of your results and one month for writing up your results and putting together presentations. If you need to spend more time than this to do a bigger survey then it might be better to spend your time preparing a submission to attract funds to employ someone to do this for you or to take over your other responsibilities while you continue with your survey.

How much data could you collect in a month? If you are conducting face-to-face interviews you would probably be able to complete 5 or 6 a day (assuming interviews last 45 to 60 minutes) and that will be tiring enough, but you would also have to add travel time to this if needed. This amounts to 100 to 120 interviews in total, which is quite a lot and in many cases this is likely to be in excess of what your situation

Table 12. *A comparison of three modes of data collection.*

	Mail	Telephone	Face to face
Cost	cheapest method per respondent	low to medium cost per respondent	most expensive method per respondent
Coverage	can reach a widely scattered sample	can reach a widely scattered sample, but only those with phones	depends on personal contact
Response Rate	lowest, especially with groups of low socioeconomic status	medium response rate	highest response rate
Standardization	standardized	standardization depends on the interviewer	standardization depends on the interviewer
Privacy for asking sensitive questions	good, least likely to cause embarrassment	some 'anonymity' for giving replies	may be difficult
Probing	does not permit clarification, misunderstanding will go undetected	allows for probing, reduces misunderstanding and missing answers	allows for probing, reduces misunderstanding and missing answers
Literacy	requires literacy	not restricted by literacy but language skills important	not restricted by literacy but language skills still important
Observation	no observation possible	listen to respondent	listen to and watch respondent

requires, especially as you will have to analyse all the results as well! Of course, if you spent a month sending out mailed questionnaires you could have thousands in your sample, but again you must confine yourself to what you can analyse. Chances are you will tire quickly if you attempt to collect data personally for more than a month at the rate we have advised. You could split the task with a colleague and conserve your energies!

What other resources should you consider? You must have clerical assistance for typing drafts of your questionnaire and for the typing of your report. You need facilities for duplicating copies of your questionnaire. If you are to share the workload with others for an interviewer-administered survey, you will need to undergo training sessions to make sure that all parties are familiar with the procedures and conduct the interviews in a similar fashion. For mailed surveys an often forgot-

ten cost is postage, including postage for reply-paid envelopes for respondents to return their completed questionnaires. If you are holding
public meetings to present your results, you will need to make sure
that you have allocated funds to cover advertising, venue hire, refreshments and so on. You may also need to cover the costs of printing and
distribution of your report.

The Questionnaire

The questionnaire is the form you use to record the data you are collecting. It is also called the *survey instrument*. It may be an interview
schedule, in which case you are the person who reads it and you record
what respondents say in reply to your questions. Alternatively, it could
be a self-completed questionnaire in which case your respondents read
the questions and fill out their answers. In the latter case you may need
to be extra careful about the design and format of your questionnaire
to make it attractive and easy to answer.

With structured methods of investigation, the aim is to construct the
content and sequence of questions in such a way as to encourage completion of the questionnaire with a high degree of accuracy. A great
deal of time is spent in getting the questions right and then, with interview situations, making sure that the person administering the questionnaire sticks to the precise wording.

There is a reason for this. Your questionnaire is trying to find out
things about your population, what they think, what they believe, how
they behave and so on. When your start to detect differences and patterns in the replies you are getting from your respondents you want to
be sure that these are true reflections of real differences between individuals and not just artifacts produced by variations in the way a
question was put to them. Consider for example the question: 'Are you
likely to give up smoking in the next month?'. The reply you will get
to this question will probably differ from the reply you will get to a
similar question: 'So, are you really likely to give up smoking in the
next month?' The attempt to make sure that all respondents are presented with the same series of questions is called *standardization*.

Broad question areas

The first step is to write down the broad areas you wish to cover in
your questionnaire. These dimensions may have been determined by
you in earlier qualitative approaches or you may be using other guides
according to the reading and consulting you may have done in relation
to the topic. Don't turn these into questions just yet. The point at this
stage is to make sure that you have covered the topic area adequately.
Don't forget to include sociodemographic information such as age, sex
and ethnic status and other factors about the respondent that may be
of interest.

Wording and format of questions

Think about what you are trying to measure or record in your questionnaire. Knowledge? Attitude? Beliefs? Characteristics? Behaviour? This will determine the style of your approach. For example, in assessing knowledge it is common to provide formats such as true/false responses to statements or selecting items from a list of alternatives. In assessing attitudes, it is common to make statements and ask respondents to nominate whether they agree or disagree with the statement (see Chapter 6).

These are examples of *closed-ended questions*. These are questions followed by a list of answers and a format for making an answer. Some examples are below.

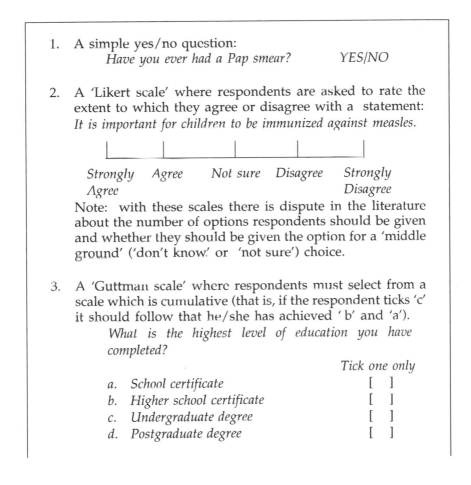

1. A simple yes/no question:
    Have you ever had a Pap smear?   *YES/NO*

2. A 'Likert scale' where respondents are asked to rate the extent to which they agree or disagree with a statement:
    It is important for children to be immunized against measles.

    Strongly   Agree   Not sure   Disagree   Strongly
    Agree   Disagree

    Note: with these scales there is dispute in the literature about the number of options respondents should be given and whether they should be given the option for a 'middle ground' ('don't know' or 'not sure') choice.

3. A 'Guttman scale' where respondents must select from a scale which is cumulative (that is, if the respondent ticks 'c' it should follow that he/she has achieved ' b' and 'a').
    What is the highest level of education you have completed?
                                                          Tick one only
    a.   *School certificate*   [   ]
    b.   *Higher school certificate*   [   ]
    c.   *Undergraduate degree*   [   ]
    d.   *Postgraduate degree*   [   ]

4. A multiple-choice question, where the respondent must choose just one answer.
    Which of one of the following is the most likely to be a method of transmission of the AIDS virus?

		Tick one only
a.	*Sharing kitchen utensils*	[ ]
b.	*Sharing needles*	[ ]
c.	*Toilet seats*	[ ]

5. A multiple choice format which allows multiple responses.
    Which of the following symptoms have you experienced in the past month?

		You may tick more than one
a.	*Headache*	[ ]
b.	*Dizziness*	[ ]
c.	*Fever*	[ ]
d.	*Vomiting*	[ ]
e.	*Inability to sleep*	[ ]
f.	*Skin rashes*	[ ]
g.	*Shortness of breath*	[ ]

6. A rank order, in which respondents are asked to put items in order of importance.
    Please number the following health problems in your community in order of importance. Place a 1 next to the problem which you think is the most important. Place a 2 next to the problem which you think is the next most important and so on through to 5 for the problem of least importance.

Alcohol and drug dependence	[ ]
Loneliness and depression	[ ]
Motor vehicle accidents	[ ]
Pollution	[ ]
Industrial accidents	[ ]

In contrast, with open-ended questions the nature of the answer given is left entirely to the respondent. An example of an open-ended question is: 'What things do you think you could do to protect yourself from the risk of catching the AIDS virus?' As mentioned previously, open-ended questions generate a wide range of replies and they are frequently used in the beginning of an investigation to 'map out' prevailing knowledge, attitudes and so on as the basis for designing closed-ended questions.

It is important to take care in the wording of questions. This applies to both open and closed-ended questions. Firstly, the language you use should suit your respondents. This is particularly important for health and medical terms as we often forget that many people are not familiar with them. Secondly, you must ensure that your questions are clear and specific. The question: 'Have you seen a doctor recently? (yes/no)' is too vague. It would be better rephrased as 'Have you been to see a doctor in the last week?' or 'How many times have you been to see a doctor in the last month?' Avoid double questions such as 'Do you prefer to be cared for by female doctors and female nurses? (yes/no).' (What happens if they prefer one and don't mind about the other?) Avoid double negatives in questions and make sure questions are not ambiguous. Also, avoid questions that are too ambitious such as: 'Rank the following 25 factors in order of importance . . . '! Biased or leading questions may be subtle. Consider, for example, the following:

How often do you have sex with other men?
(Presupposes that the respondent does have sex with other men; only appropriate if this follows a question that establishes this.)

How do you think the government should look after the health needs of women, by providing special services or what?
(The question supplies just one of many possible alternatives. It may be easier for the respondent to just agree with the suggestion that has been given than to consider the additional options.)

It is important to take special care in the wording of *sensitive questions*, such as questions that reveal a person's 'status' (income, education, occupation and so on) and questions regarding behaviour or attitudes that respondents fear others may not approve of. It is often a good idea to preface such questions with a statement which 'gives permission' for a respondent to give a certain type of response. For example, in trying to get people to admit that they do not always take the amount of medication a doctor has prescribed, it has been shown that 'non-compliers' are more likely to reveal themselves if the question starts with a statement to create the sort of climate where they will feel comfortable.[2] For example: 'Some people find that there are occasions when they do not take all of their medications . . . ' The questions that follow would then ask about this. Note that it is important not to take this so far that the question is biased, and people who are good compliers feel that they are missing out on something!

Another way to make respondents comfortable about replying to sensitive questions and give you accurate replies is to make sure that the question format does not require people to place themselves in the extreme boundaries. For example, a person who drinks on average, say, 10 glasses of beer a day will feel more comfortable if their reply to your question looks like this . . .

a.   *2 or less drinks per day*   [ ]
b.   *3–5 drinks per day*   [ ]
c.   *6–8 drinks per day*   [ ]
d.   *9–11 drinks per day*   [√]
e.   *12–14 drinks per day*   [ ]
f.   *15 or more*   [ ]

. . . than if their reply to your question looks like this:

a.   *2 or less*   [ ]
b.   *3–5 drinks per day*   [ ]
c.   *6–9 drinks per day*   [ ]
d.   *10 or more*   [√]

With sensitive questions in an interview situation, it has also been found that people will feel more comfortable replying to your question if they can look down at a card handed to them and simply nominate that they are, for example, in income category 'b' than if you make them have to say '$25 000 per year'.

Question sequence

Now that you have your questions, they should be put into order. Firstly, pay attention to any logical sequence (like asking about family size and children's ages before you inquire about use of childcare services). You should insert *filter questions* to prevent some groups of respondents being asked questions that are inappropriate, for example, non-smokers being asked about the number of cigarettes per day. A filter question would be 'Do you smoke cigarettes? (Yes/No If 'no', go to Question 13)'.

Start the questionnaire with fairly innocuous questions which are easy to answer to get a bit of a rhythm going. Leave sensitive, threatening or difficult questions until the end. They are more likely to be answered once your respondent has been through your other questions and feels more secure. Sometimes, no matter how well you think you have worded your question, a respondent may choose not to answer. That is also why it is good to have these questions towards the end: if they are at the beginning, the respondent may then decide to skip some of your other questions as well!

When your questionnaire is long you should insert *transition statements* between sections. A transition statement simply informs the respondent what the next series of questions is going to cover. This helps to promote interest and cooperation, particularly if you also take the opportunity to remind the respondent of the purpose of the questions.

An example of a transition statement would be: 'Now I am going to ask you about your leisure activites on weekends. This will help us to plan better facilities for families in this area.

Layout and appearance

First of all you need to scan your questionnaire and make sure that respondents can see each question clearly and where they should put their answers or replies. For example, you could line questions up so that all the respondents' answers are on the right hand side. That way it is easy to spot where an answer has not been given. Place adequate space between questions and don't make the mistake of crowding as much as you can onto a page to try to make the questionnaire look shorter! People will fill out a well set out questionnaire of several pages in length with more enthusiasm than they will tackle something that is confusing because it is all bunched up, with little room for their replies.

For a self-completed questionnaire, endeavour to make the questionnaire as attractive as possible. Pay attention to paper quality, the print style and size, the colour of the paper and so on. You could even include graphics. It is better to have questions placed on one side of the paper only, as people often accidently skip questions on the verso of a double-sided questionnaire which is stapled in the top left-hand corner only. However, to save paper you could have questions typed on both sides provided that you go to the extra trouble of making the questionnaire into a 'book' with a number of centre staples. This way the questionnaire folds out so that all questions are easily seen.

At the top of the front page of the questionnaire don't forget to put *identifiers*, which are the data that can tell you at a glance important information about the respondent. For example, this might include the respondent's number in the study (allocated to them by you), perhaps a code for the suburb or the school, a code number for the person who interviewed them (if it has not all been done by yourself) and so on.

Cover letter and introduction

You need to put together a covering letter to accompany your self-completed questionnaire. The content of this will be much the same as what you would cover in the introductory remarks in an interviewer-based survey. The purpose of your covering letter is to interest respondents in your survey and persuade them to participate. Some of the points you may wish to cover are as follows:[3]

- the importance of the survey
- the importance of the respondent's participation
- the importance of the respondent's participation even if they feel not qualified to answer all questions
- how the respondent may benefit from the research

- how long it will take to complete the questionnaire
- how easy it will be to complete the questionnaire
- how the respondent was selected
- that replies are kept confidential
- offer for feedback of results
- note of urgency
- your credibility or the importance of your organization
- your appreciation
- contact person for enquiries or further information.

Of course, you have to make sure that you can stand by all the assurances you have made! Try also to keep the length to a minimum.

Pilotting the questionnaire

When your questionnaire is in final form, circulate it among friends and colleagues to get their opinion. Ask them to try to fill it out. Ask them what they think of your covering letter as well. This initial consultation is crucial because chances are you have been so involved with the design of your questionnaire over the past week or so that you have lost your critical perspective. After you have redrafted your questionnaire, incorporating modifications and suggestions that you might have received, it is time to try the questionnaire out with 'real' respondents.

Select 5 or 6 people initially (it doesn't matter too much at this stage how you select them). Explain the project you are doing and ask them to help you by filling out your questionnaire and then agreeing to talk with you about it. Then, with the completed questionnaire in front of you, you should go through each question trying to see how well it was understood and whether the response formats were adequate. Also ask about the question sequence, whether the form looked attractive, if there was anything offensive in the content or presentation, was it easy to read, did it leave out things they thought were important and so on. At the end of these interviews you should revise and retest the questionnaire, talking to some of the original respondents (to check that you interpreted them correctly) and with a new group.

How many people should be in your pilot study? There are no rules about this and really you should continue to test your instrument until you are satisfied with it. As a rough guide, your pilot group would be roughly equivalent to 10% to 20% of the number in your main study. You won't be able to 'recycle' participants from your pilot into your main study if you suspect that the experience will change the way in which they will answer your questions.

In the pilot survey you also conduct a trial run of your *data manage-*

ment and *data analysis*. Data management refers to the procedure you put into place to keep track of respondents in your study and check the quality of the data that is being collected (such as, the proportion of missing answers, answers that don't make sense, and so on). In large-scale surveys a full-time data manager may be appointed. For your purpose you need to check the quality of responses as they come in and keep a log of what is happening in the study (when questionnaires were sent out, date received, date reminders sent to respondents who have not yet replied and so on). If you are having someone else analyse your data you will also need to keep a record of the number and so on.

A trial run of the data analysis is conducted to make sure that the questionnaire is going to produce data you can make sense of. It is also a good way of making sure that your questionnaire has left nothing out. Working backwards from the sorts of things you want your data to say will also tell you if your questionnaire has collected more data than you are interested in. This is a common error, and spotting it now will allow you to eliminate some questions and shorten the questionnaire.

Response rates

Your response rate is the number of questionnaires returned to you compared with the number of questionnaires you sent out. This proportion is usually expressed as a percentage and you should generally aim to get 65% or better. There is a reason for this.

The people who respond to invitations to cooperate with a survey are generally different from those people who refuse. If a large proportion of people refuse to participate in your survey then you cannot place much faith in the answers of the few people who do participate as these are likely to be an unrepresentative group. It is not always easy to predict which way the bias might be. For example, the sort of people who respond to your follow-up survey of participants in a quit smoking programme may be the ones who have managed to stay off cigarettes and are pleased for the opportunity to 'register' their success. On the other hand, your group of respondents may instead be largely comprised of people who are still smoking and want to tell you that your programme is awful!

Even with a good response rate you may still get some bias in your results if a particular type of person refused to participate. To get an insight into this you can follow up non-respondents and see if they will give you just a little information about themselves, such as sociodemographic characteristics which you can compare with your responders. Another technique is to compare the sorts of replies you got back from successive waves of late responders with the sorts of replies you received from people who responded on time. This will tell you if the less-interested people are more likely, for example, to be still smoking or whatever. With relatively small sample sizes, unfortunately, it may be hard to spot differences between these groups.

Most researchers will tell you that response rate is important no matter what the total number of respondents is. It is quite different and far better to get back 120 questionnaires from a random sample of 130 (92% response rate) than it is to get back 120 when you sent out 250 (48% response rate). Because of this, rather than spending a lot of energy trying to get your questionnaire to a great many people, you should concentrate on getting it back, completed, from a smaller number of people. To do this you can send out reminders, second copies of the questionnaires and so on.

The Analysis

Making sense of qualitative data

Qualitative data may be recorded in a number of different ways such as video tapes, audio tapes and, most commonly, written notes. If you have been conducting focus groups you will find it difficult to get by without a tape of the proceedings. The first step is to simply *organize* your data and put it into working order. Tapes have to be transcribed in full or summarized.

You can begin to put different types of information into separate files and work out an index system to help you retrieve this easily. For example, everything people said about the problems of social isolation could go into one pile, everything they said about alcohol abuse could go into another pile and so on. If you can't physically separate these responses from each other (because they are written on the same piece of paper) you can start to code these responses instead. For example everything about alcohol abuse gets an 'A' or a '1', everything about social isolation gets a '2' and so on. As you are reading, if you discover mention of a different type of problem, say, teenage crime, that would get a '3'. You are not going to do numerical manipulations with these numbers, they are simply your coding categories which later will make patterns in your data easier to recognize. As you work through the data, building up *coding categories*, you should also enter these into a coding manual to keep track of what your codes mean. At this stage, when in doubt about the separateness of a new problem or idea, give it a code number. Merging of categories, if appropriate, will come later. You should work through until all the data in each interview has been coded.

The next step is *shaping*, which is looking for sweeping patterns and themes in the data. Are some categories associated or linked together? For example, do the people who are concerned about teenage crime link it with concerns about social isolation? Is there another group of

Figure 24.

Room too stuffy and crowded, venue ||

Group leader's superior attitude |||| |||| |||

Film on childrearing |||

Too much talk about mother's role not father's |||

Nothing, I enjoyed it. I liked it all ||||

Not enough time for discussion |||

No childcare facilities ||

Other people allowed to talk too much ||

Group leader not able to control discussion |||| ||||

respondents nominating environmental concerns? What are the other interests of this group? Can you really consider them to be a separate group? Why? Many researchers encourage their colleagues to also inspect their data to verify the patterns that are emerging or offer alternative ways of interpreting what is going on.

Explaining is the third step. Here you really want to understand and interpret what the data are saying. Look carefully for information that contradicts your first conclusion. For example, let's say that most people said that they supported the idea of more drug education programmes ... but that a lot of people did not list drugs as a priority. This may not seem to make sense, but maybe people believe that they should simply be given as many services as possible. Don't force a conclusion or a rationalization on the data. Don't presuppose that all the data set will be consistent. That is why your original coding system is important, you and others can go back to reread and reassess the conclusions that you draw.

Analysis of qualitative data is time-consuming and it requires a high degree of skill. It is also very rewarding as you can use your respondents' own words to identify and explain your results. On many occasions, however, you will not be transcribing hour-long unstructured interviews and building up your entire data set from this basis. Often you will simply be analysing the responses to a single open-ended question from a self-completed questionnaire. How should you go about this?

The principles here are much the same. A common practice is to do something like a long-hand version of what researchers call 'factor analysis' which is done on a computer. Let's say that your question was 'What did you like least about the programme?' Take the first questionnaire and write down what your respondent said. Let's say it was 'The room was too stuffy and crowded. Superior attitude of group leader'. Put these underneath each other on the left hand side of a blank page. Then take the next questionnaire and read the respondent's answer to the same question. Let's say that they said: 'Venue. The film on child-rearing'. Because 'venue' is a bit like what the first person also mentioned, you would write this up next to the first person's words about the room and mark next to it to indicate that two people had now said this. The comment about the film is a new idea so it gets listed on its own, still on the left hand side, beneath the others. You then pick up the third person's questionnaire. Let's say that they said 'Group leader'. You can see that you start to build up a picture of the most common (negative) feelings about your programme and your analysis sheet could end up looking something like Figure 24.

This gives you a clear idea of the most common responses. A reasonable analysis of this question would be:

> Although a few respondents could not nominate anything they didn't like about the programme, the most common problem that participants mentioned was the group leaders. This mostly concerned what participants described as their 'superior attitude', but also included criticism of their capacity to control discussion and allow more people to contribute. Others things participants noted were the limitations of the venue and facilities (the small room, no childcare facilities), the film and an overemphasis on the role of the mother (as opposed to the role of the father).

Note that you cannot subject this data to quantitative manipulation. You cannot say, for example, that 60% of people disliked the venue or 12% hated the film. This is because a summary of this nature carries the implication that respondents were given an opportunity to comment on each of these aspects in turn (such as in a list with a 'Yes/No' response format). If someone fails to mention something you don't know if they thought of it and then discounted its importance, or whether they failed to think of it at all. In fact, they generated the response categories themselves. The tally marks are purely to help you identify general trends. To prevent errors of this nature a lot of people conduct this sort of analysis without tally marks.

Making sense of quantitative data

The way in which you analyse quantitative data depends on the scale of measurement you provided for recording answers for each question of the questionnaire. That is, it depends on what the numbers really refer to in the answers on your completed forms

For example, in some questions the answer '1' may be a code for a female and '2' may be the code for male. In another question '1' may refer to the number of times the respondent has visited a GP since discharge from hospital. In the latter case the '1' really has a quantitative property. It is half of two, for example, so someone who has answered '2' for this question has been to a GP twice as much as the first respondent who answered '1'. It is important to note that the numbers refer to very different types of things here and not get mixed up. For the first question on gender, for example, all you can do is add up your males and female, but quantitatively you can't get away with saying that a female is worth two males! However, when you are using the same numbers to refer to doctor visits, you can say that one respondent has used services more and you can go on to do further quantitative manipulations like working out the average number of visits by respondents to doctors in your sample. Therefore, the way in which you approach the analysis of each question will vary.

For questions that list things like people's sex, marital status, and whether their child is immunized against measles (yes/no) the scale of measurement is called *nominal* and the type of data you have collected is *categorial*. It is a scale of measurement which puts people into categories. The number of categories doesn't matter. You could have two, such as with sex, or you could have more, such as when you divide the population up into smokers, ex-smokers, and people who have never smoked. The number allocated to describe that category is for coding purposes only and has no quantitative properties. The only way to analyse this data is to count the number of people in each category and turn these into *proportions or percentages*. So you would refer to the proportion of people in the sample who were women, or the proportion who could list correctly the ways in which AIDS is transmitted and so on.

The next scale of measurement is called the *ordinal* scale. This is like when you ask people to rank problems or factors in order of importance, say rating the importance of factors that contribute to the quality of life for cancer patients. Let's assume that the example below represents one respondent's answer. A ranking of 1 represents most important, 2 is next most important and so on:

Being pain free	[1]
Being in a pleasant enviroment	[4]
Having a good relationship with spouse	[2]
Religious conviction	[5]
Access to caring medical care	[3]

Although the respondent ranked being pain free as 1 and religious conviction as 5, you cannot say that religious conviction is 5 times less important. Neither can you say that having a good relationship with a spouse is half as important as being pain free. The numbers themselves cannot be subjected to quantitative manipulation in this way. The magnitude between each number has no meaning. All the numbers do is reveal the order of importance. The respondent could have revealed their order of importance even if you had instructed them to rank them differently (i.e., with 5 being the most important).

How would you summarize the data from this question from a group of, say, 20 respondents? One simple way to do this would be to take each factor and add up all the 'scores' given to this factor from each respondent and then divide by 20, giving you an average or *mean*. You could do this for each factor and then construct a group ranking on the basis of these by putting them in order from the smallest average 'score' to the highest. Again, you are not interested in the size of difference between each factor, just the order from smallest (most important) to biggest (least important).

However, consider the situation where most people rank being pain free as 1, but enough people rank it as a 5 to pull its overall score down to second most important or even perhaps third most important. In these circumstances your analysis may convey more meaning if you report on the proportion of people who ranked being pain free as 1, the proportion of people who ranked access to medical care as 1 and so on. In this way you are really only highlighting the first ranking and treating the data as if it were categorical. You really must leave this sort of decision until you have inspected the data in front of you.

What about questions such as : 'What is your age?' or 'What is your weight?' or 'How many people are in your family?' The answer to this is a number and this number is able to be subjected to quantitative manipulation. The scale of measurement is called the *interval* scale. The numbers on this scale do have relationships to each other . . . so you can comfortably (at last!) say that if someone writes 3 next to family size, then this family is half the size of that belonging to a respondent who has put 6 as their answer to this question. With this sort of data you can summarize responses from your sample into *means*. You should also calculate standard deviations. A *standard deviation* is simply an indication of the variation in the scores. If you are familiar with these terms then you should find out the formulae for these calculations from an elementary statistical textbook. If this is the first time you have heard of these terms then it would be wiser to ask a statistician or someone else skilled in statistical methods to explain more about it.

Let's consider how you would analyse data from a Likert scale, where you might be assessing the extent to which the respondents in your sample agree or disagree with a statement such as in the following example.

'People are largely responsible for their own health'

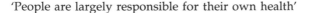
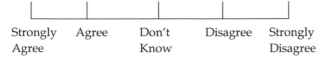

| Strongly | Agree | Don't | Disagree | Strongly |
| Agree | | Know | | Disagree |

Some people would argue that you can treat data that has been derived from a Likert scale as if it is in the interval scale of measurement. That is, like with ages or number of children in a family, the interval between items in the scales are the same. So, as the difference between age 4 and age 5 is the same as the difference between age 5 and age 6, so they would argue that the difference between 'strongly agree' and 'agree' is the same as the difference between 'disagree' and 'strongly disagree'. You would then assign numerical values to these. So you could assign 2 to 'strongly agree', 1 to 'agree', 0 to don't know, -1 to 'disagree' and -2 to 'strongly disagree'. You could then proceed to analyse the data in the normal way (that is, calculate an agreement 'score' for each person and go on to calculate a 'mean agreement score' for the whole group). Other quantitative manipulations are also possible and these get more complicated and more the province of statisticians and psychometricians.

On the other hand, some people would argue that 'strongly agree' and 'agree' mean different things to different people and this is essentially qualitative data put into different categories. In this way what you have is no more than proportions of people who fall into these categories which you would report in the same way as you do for all categorical data, that is with percentages. Your analysis could for example look like the following:

Agreement and disagreement with the statement: 'People are largely responsible for their own health'

	% of respondents
Strongly agree	7
Agree	25
Don't know/not sure	12
Disagree	40
Strongly disagree	16

For descriptive purposes, probably the second approach is more illuminating.

With all the approaches discussed above it would be possible to conduct an analysis of subgroups within your sample, and this may reveal patterns disguised by the overall means and frequencies. For example, are people with a higher socioeconomic status more likely to say that they agree with the statement about self-responsibility for health? Do female cancer patients consider different factors to be more important for quality of life than male cancer patients? However, within the confines of a small sample size you are unlikely to have the 'statistical power' to pick up some of these differences. Again, if ascertaining this sort of information is crucial to your study and the development of your intervention, you should channel your energies into securing funding for additional resources to carry out this work. The data from the survey you have conducted may indicate some of these trends and should be used as the basis of your submission.

The Report

At last, at the end of your analysis you should still have about one quarter of the total time you allocated to your survey for the writing up of your results. This emphasis is not out of proportion. In applied fields such as health promotion, your survey is only really as good as the sorts of planning decisions and interventions that grow from it and this depends on how well you can communicate your results. Remember that you should have different strategies to reach different groups with your information. Many health workers produce a formal report and a more friendly looking pamphlet or booklet that can be distributed in the community. Another approach is to make a slide tape programme that can be part of a static display. This would include 'action shots' of the survey in progress, some of the different people involved (the survey team) and so on as well as your results, displayed in pictorial form. This is particularly important when you have involved members of the community or the target group in the conduct of the survey as it gives obvious recognition to their efforts.

In this section we will outline simply what should be covered in your formal report.

Summary
A brief overview of the problem, the survey methods and the main findings of the survey. Lots of people only read this section so it is important that you include important major findings and recommendations. Although it comes first, it is often in practice much easier to write the summary last.

Background
This functions as the introduction and statement of the problem. It should give the rationale for the conduct of the survey and mention any reports or references that are relevant that you may have discovered in your earlier literature review. At the end of this section the reader should be persuaded of the importance of the problem being investigated. This creates interest in the sections to follow.

Method

Describe your survey subjects, how they were selected, the survey questions, what method you used in the survey to collect information (self-completed questionnaires, etc.), and the main topics covered in the questionnaire.

Results

Firstly report your response rate and make comments about the extent to which any problems in this area might affect the interpretation of your findings. Group the results according to topics or present them in a logical sequence (not necessarily the order of questions on the questionnaire). It is usually best to start with the sociodemographic and other data that describe your respondents. Use graphs, tables, pie charts, etc. to illustrate your findings and make them easier to read and understand.

Discussion and Conclusions

This is where you comment on your results and introduce some interpretation and explanation. A common strategy is to punctuate the summary of quantitative data with quotations from your qualitative investigation. Also point out where there is conflict in the data, where say the quantitative and qualitative data don't agree. Don't force reasons for this if nothing is obvious to you. The purpose of distributing your report and presenting it to other people is also to stimulate discussion and interpretation. Comment on how your findings confirm or differ from those of other investigators. Draw conclusions from the data and relate these back to your original statement of the problem.

Recommendations

If you are in a position to make recommendations from your survey do so. It is also common to delay the writing of this section until there has been discussion of the report.

References

List the full reference (author, title, year, volume, pages, journal or publisher) of any other person's work which you cite.

Appendices

Include a copy of your questionnaire, covering letter and any other background material you feel should be included (such as press releases).

References

1. Barrera M. Social support in the adjustment of pregnant adolescents: assessment issues. In: Gottlieb, BH. (ed.) *Social Networks and Social Support.* Beverly Hills: Sage Publications, 1981; 69–96.
2. Dunbar J. Issues in assessment. In: Cohen SJ (ed.) *New Directions in Patient Compliance.* Massachusetts: Lexington Books, 1979.
3. Erdos P. *Professional Mail Surveys.* Melbourne, Florida: Krieger, 1983.

Further Reading

Sudman D, Bradburn NM *Asking Questions. A Practical Guide to Questionnaire Design.* San Francisco: Jossey Bass, 1986.

Abramson JH. *Survey Methods in Community Medicine.* Edinburgh: Churchill Livingston, 1979.

Miles MB, Huberman AM. *Qualitative Data Analysis. A Sourcebook of New Methods.* Beverly Hills: Sage Publications, 1982.

Chapter 8

HOW TO DO A
LITERATURE REVIEW

OBJECTIVES

At the end of this chapter you should be able to:

1. Access literature relevant to your field of interest.
2. Critically appraise the articles you find.
3. Evaluate interventions and programmes reported in the literature and compare their relative success.
4. Explain how you can use other people's research findings in your own needs assessment or programme planning or in the evaluation of your programme's effects.

Looking at the research literature can be a daunting process. First you have to find it: this can be a time-consuming and frustrating exercise. Once you have found it, you feel obliged to read it. And then you feel obliged to find more literature. Struggling with jargon and terms that you are unfamiliar with can slow your reading down. Once you have read each article you need to make a number of decisions: can you accept these findings as true, can you apply these findings to your own research, and whom do you believe when different authors find contradictory results?

With all those obstacles, why bother to look at the research literature?

Why? Because the work of previous researchers can help shape your own research and programme planning. Not only can it make you more aware of what has been done, it can also provide you with a framework of how others have gone about exploring the same area that you are interested in and what the main issues are.

Before we go any further, a few definitions and disclaimers.

157

This chapter is intended mainly for people who have not had the need or opportunity to carry out a literature review. It therefore assumes little knowledge about large university libraries and how to use them, so a lot of this will be familiar ground for some readers.

Reasons for Consulting the Research Literature

When you begin to search for literature it is important that you are aware of why you are conducting the search and what you are trying to find in the literature. Within the field of evaluation you will probably be looking in the literature for one or both of these reasons:

- to find out about a particular health issue or target group to give direction to your own needs assessment work;
- to see whether a particular type of intervention or programme works, in order to direct programme planning and implementation.

Your reason for looking at the literature will influence what you look for in an article and what you do with it. The way into the literature is much the same, though, so first we'll discuss how to find it, then we'll look at how to read and appraise the literature in light of your purpose.

A third reason for consulting the literature is to find a measurement instrument to use for either process, impact or outcome evaluation. This chapter will get you started on finding journals and articles relevant to your field, but for a more detailed look at finding measures, see Chapter 10.

Finding Research Literature

There are a number of different ways you can start a literature search. Not all of these are equally efficient.

Research literature is most commonly published in journals (or periodicals), less often in books. Where do you find journals? University, hospital or large college libraries are the most likely places to look for journals. Once at the library, there are four ways to go about finding your research literature. In increasing order of sophistication they are: (i) random perusal of (relevant) journals; (ii) subject catalogue; (iii) indexes and abstracts; and (iv) computer searches.

As an example, if you were planning to run stop smoking groups it is likely that relevant articles would appear in health education journals, medical journals and behavioural science journals. After locating these journals on the shelves, you could search through the contents page to locate suitable material. Using this method you will probably find some articles. However, this method is random, it will take you a long time, and you will probably miss some good articles that have been published in other journals you are not aware of.

Subject catalogue

You could go to the subject catalogue and look up smoking. What you are most likely to find are books on what smoking does to your health; books presenting the wider social and political context of the cigarette manufacturing and sales industry; cigarette use in particular societies; and books summarizing anti-smoking efforts over the last 10 years.

Books which summarize research over a period of time can provide a useful introduction to your subject area. However information printed in books is usually general, likely to be several years old, and may not be research-based. Research-based information provides you with specific information about how a programme was planned, implemented and evaluated with a specific target group.

Subject catalogues are not very useful for finding journals or journal articles appropriate to your area. Obviously you need to look elsewhere for the sort of information that you will need to plan or evaluate your own programme.

Abstracts and indexes

There are a number of services which collate and publish abstracts (summaries) of articles relevant to a particular field or profession (e.g. *Psychological Abstracts*). The abstracts are further organized under subject headings (e.g. attitudes, substance abuse) and collated in volumes according to the year the articles appeared in print. Each entry includes a reference code for finding the article. You can preview articles by reading their abstracts first, then decide whether you need to get the entire article.

In some fields a similar services is provided which indexes relevant articles by their titles (or shortened titles) but does not include abstracts (e.g. *Index Medicus*).

Abstracts and indexes are usually housed in the reference section of the library and are available for use by students and members of the public at any time during library hours. You don't need to book but you will probably need to ask a reference librarian to direct you to the abstracts for your particular area of interest if you haven't used them before. Write down the names and the call numbers (the number on each book in a library which tells you where it can be found) for next time.

Useful abstracts and indexes for health promotion include:

- *Index Medicus* (medical journals)
- *Psychological Abstracts*
- *Sociological Abstracts*
- *ERIC* (Educational Resources Information Center)

- *Social Sciences Citation Index*
- *Current Contents*: Clinical Practice
                       Life Sciences
                       Social and Behavioural Sciences
- *FAMILY* (Family Medicine Literature Index)
- *APAIS* (Australian Public Affairs Information Service) contains newspaper and magazine articles which can also be useful
- Don't forget *HEAPS* for reports on current programmes being run in your field.

Let's say you are going to look in *Psychological Abstracts* for articles on smoking cessation. This publication includes so many references that it has to be split up into different sections. When you get to the *Psychological Abstracts* on the shelf you will find rows and rows of volumes with this title.

Start with the most recent cumulative subject index—this gives you a list of articles published over the last three years, organized under subject headings, or the most recent year's subject index (e.g. 1989 M–Z).

You might look under 'S' for 'smoking', or under 'T' for 'tobacco use'. Then you might find some under 'H' for 'health education' about smoking; some under 'W' for 'women's health and smoking' etc. It all depends on the angle you're looking for and on the way the subjects are organized in the index. You might need to check the range of headings within the abstracts index to work out which of them cover the concepts you have in mind.

In *Psychological Abstracts* what you will find at this stage is a couple of short descriptive phrases about each article (not necessarily the title and not the abstract) and a code number. Write down all the code numbers for the articles that sound promising. You then look up each number in the next set of volumes which have the year, and the code numbers they cover, printed on the outside (e.g. 1989 20595 - 36112). Next to the code number is printed the abstract and a reference to where you can look up and read the whole article.

Again you select those which still sound relevant to your study and discard those which, from the abstract, are clearly outside your area of interest. Write down the *whole reference* (include author(s), title of article, name of the journal, date, year, page) so that if you can't find the article immediately you have enough information to look it up later or at another library.

These steps are slightly different for indexes. If you are using *Index Medicus*, your first step of looking at the latest subject index is the same, but instead of finding a description and a code number, you get the

Figure 25 *An example from* Psychological Abstracts *subject index.*

Tobacco Smoking
ability to self cure obesity & smoking behavior, 22–80 yr old faculty & graduate students & university support staff, partial replication of study by S. Schachter, 16432

abstinence from tobacco, withdrawal symptoms, 19–63 yr old tobacco smokers, 5323

agreement between self report vs laboratory tests of alcohol & tobacco & caffeine & marihuana & other drug usage, mothers tested at 2 & 4 mo postpartum, 7141

alcohol & drug & cigarette use patterns, 21-24 yr olds initially surveyed as 7th–9th graders, 8-yr longitudinal study, 27872

alveolar carbon monoxide validation of smoking rates, treatment success & misreporting of abstinence, volunteer smokers in behavioral smoking cessation clinics, 32516

anti-smoking counseling practices & success, family practice physicians, 35715 } *let's say you're interested in this one …*

antismoking program completion, resistance to relapse, 30–59 yr old program participants, 23136

applicability judgments of smoking attributes, college student smokers vs nonsmokers, 30314

Figure 26. Psychological Abstracts, *abstracts volume.*

35714. Courtwright, David T. (U Harford) Charles Terry, *The Opium Problem*, and American narcotic policy. *Journal of Drug Issues*, 1986 (Sum), Vol 16(3), 421-434.—Presents a biographical sketch of Charles Edward Terry (1878–1945), a public health reformer who pioneered narcotic maintenance and coauthored *The Opium Problem* (1982). Terry's career and ideas are described against the background of the Harrison Act and the formation of American narcotic policy, against which Terry vigorously, but unsuccessfully, dissented.

35715. Commings, K Michael; Giovino, Gary; Emont, Seth L.; Sciandra, Roswell et al. (Roswell Park Memorial Inst, Dept of Cancer Control & Epidemiology, Buffalo, NY) Factors influencing success in counseling patients to stop smoking. *Patient Education & Counseling*. 1986(Jun), Vol 8(2), 189–200. —Examined the anti-smoking counseling practices of a group of 28 family practice physicians and related these to success in persuading 283 cigarette-smoking patients to stop smoking. Patients were followed over a 3-mo period to assess changes in smoking behavior. Findings show wide variation among physicians in the percentage of patients who tried to quit (range: 20-77%) and the percentage of patients who succeeded in quitting (range: 0–25%). Two counseling practices, advising patients to set a target date for quitting and scheduling follow-up visits with patients to monitor progress, were related to the percentage of a physician's patients who quit smoking.

now you need to find **Patient Education and Counseling** *…*

162   EVALUATING HEALTH PROMOTION

Figure 27.   *An example from* Index Medicus.

SMOKING
see related
TOBACCO USE DISORDER
Acute effects of maternal smoking on human fetal heart
function. Srensen KE, et al.
   Acta Obstet Gynecol Scand 1987; 66(3): 217–20
Factors associated with smoking behavior in adolescent
girls. Hover SJ, et al. **Addict Behav** 1988; 13(2): 139–45
Impact of smoking on heart attacks, strokes, blood pressure control, drug dose, and quality of life aspects in
the International prospective Primary Prevention
Study in Hypertension. Bühler FR, et al. **Am Heart J**
1988 Jan; 115(1 Pt 2): 282–81
The Medical Research Council Hypertension Trial: the
smoking patient. Dollery C, et al. **Am Heart J** 1988 Jan;
115(1 pt 2): 276–81
Cigarette smoking and hemostatic function. FizGerald
GA, et al. Am Heart J 1988 Jan; 115 (1 Pt 2):267–71 (34
ref.) Strategies to reduce risk factors in hypertensive
patients who smoke. Kaplan NM. **Am Heart J** 1988;
115 (1 Pt 2):288–94
The cardiovascular pathology of smoking. McGill HC Jr.
Am Heart J 1988 Jan; 115 (1 Pt 2):250–7 (39 ref.)
The need to manage risk factors of coronary heart
disease. Mancia G. **Am Heart J** 1988 Jan; 115 (1pt 2):
240–2
Lipid effects of smoking. MOD. **Am Heart J** 1988 Jan; 115
(1 Pt 2): 272–5

DRUG THERAPY
Do serotonin uptake inhibitors decrease smoking? Obser-
vations in a group of heavy drinkers. Sellers EM. et al.
   J Clin Psychopharmacol 1987 Dec; 7(6):417–20
Heavy smokers, smoking cessation, and clonidine [letter]
   JAMA 1988 Sept 16; 260(11):1552–3
Internists and nicotine gum. Cummings SR, et al. **JAMA**
1988 Sep 16; 260(11): 1565–9
Long-term use of nicotine chewing gum. Occurrence, de-
terminants, and effect on weight again. Hajek P, et al
   JAMA 1988 Sep 16; 260(11): 1593–6
Clonidine, depression, and smoking cessation. Hughes JR.
   JAMA 1988 May 20; 259(19): 2901–2
Transdermal tobacco extract reduces reported cigarette
consumption [letter] Allen DW. **Med J Aust** 1988 Sep
19; 149(6): 342
Nicotine replacement: a critical evaluation. Based on a
conference. January 21–22, 1987, Bethesda, Maryland.
   Prog Clin Biol Res 1988; 261: 1–317

ECONOMICS
The costs of employee smoking. A computer simulation of
hospital nurses. Swank RT, et al. **Arch Intern Med**
1988 Feb; 148(2):445–8
Economic aspects of tobacco use and taxation policy.
Godfrey C, et al. **Br Med J (Chin Res)** 1988 Jul 30;
297(6644): 339–43

name of each article and the full journal reference. If you want to read the article (or the abstract only) your next step is go to the journal where the article was published. With *Index Medicus* there are often sub-headings which, with the title, help define the nature of the article. You should also be aware that the wording of the full title of an article is not always exactly the same as the title in the index, or the abstract. In some cases the abstract at the beginning of an article is not exactly the same as the abstract in the abstracting service, which is often shorter.

This process of looking up a subject, finding article titles, and then reading the abstracts is called a manual literature search.

It is a systematic search and, although it will still take up a lot of your time, it will yield most of the important articles in your area of interest. Much of your success in manual literature searching will depend on your ability to anticipate the terms that might be used as headings for your particular area of interest.

Computer searches
Computer searches involve exactly the same process as manual searches, except that they use a machine-readable index of articles (a database) instead of one on paper, and they can save you time and effort. Of course you normally have to pay for that time saving.

In most cases you would need to approach the librarian with the details of the area you are working in and he or she will set up the computer search for you. You can either have the list of references and abstracts sent to you so that you can choose which articles to look up, or you can have the articles found, photocopied and sent to you. In some instances you can also have the references and abstracts recorded on a floppy disk. Then you can read them on your PC at work or at home and print out only those you think are relevant and save some paper. Always ask the librarian which of these services are offered.

You will need to specify the key terms that describe the sort of articles you are looking for, just as you would use for your own manual search. You might need to specify the database(s) you want to have searched. These are basically on-line versions of the same abstracts journals, but there are some differences so talk to the librarian about it. For example, the equivalent of *Index Medicus* on computer database is *Medline*, but this includes *Dental and Nursing Research* as well, and it provides abstracts, not just titles. The *ERIC* database is known as *Current Index of Journals in Education*. The on-line equivalent of *Psychological Abstracts* is *PsycINFO*, available through a database called *DIALOG*. Some of these systems may be available under other names.

There will be some other aspects of the search to specify, such as whether you want English language articles only, or perhaps articles with English abstracts; and how far back in time you want to search. Usually it is best to search for recent articles initially (say the past 2 to 3 years). Then you can go back and get earlier articles if necessary. Computer searches are systematic and ensure that you do not overlook important research articles, provided you understand the basis on which they work. The computer does not use intuition the way you might if you were scanning an index, and you don't get the chance to modify your key terms along the way, so you need to choose headings or key terms which are registered on the database. And you will need to provide fairly specific topic headings or subheadings to find the literature most relevant to your area.

For example, if you searched for articles published in 1989 on smoking you might find 200, of which only 10 are really useful to you. If you had searched for articles on evaluating stop-smoking programmes, you may have turned up only the 10 useful articles. A note of warning: be careful when you are authorizing someone else to search the literature, send you the articles and charge you for it. Remember that the librarian won't be as familiar with the significant points of the literature as you are. Unless you are very clear in narrowing down what you want you may end up paying for a whole lot of reading you don't want.

You may also be able to use the computer monitoring service provided by some libraries. This provides you with any new articles that have been published in your area of interest since your initial search, by using your selected key words to search the database at regular intervals as it is updated.

One important thing to note about computer searches: although they save you the time you would otherwise need to find the information, it will take time for your request to be processed, especially if the library has a lot of requests. So don't think you can leave it to the last minute just because the computer can find things quickly.

So which way is the most efficient?

It is good to remember that the computer search is always restricted to those journals and articles which are on the database already, and may not cover all the journals or indexed journals in your area of interest. For this reason, and because computers respond only to the exact term, it is a good idea to do some preliminary reading to get a feel for the area. You should check the computer search by making sure that a couple of important articles you are already aware of appear on the list it generates. If they do not, check your key terms and the journals included in the database or databases used in the search. Then supplement your computer search with an occasional browse through current issues of relevant journals. Yes—the most efficient way is a combination of well-planned computer searches and keeping up with some journals.

From both manual and on-line searches, the abstracts will direct you to the published articles. For each article take note of: the author or authors; the title of the article; the name of the journal in which it was published; the edition (volume, year; or month, year etc.); and the page numbers.

Then you will need to go back to the library's main catalogue (the author/title catalogue or the periodicals catalogue (also called the serials list) in order to find out if the library holds the journal you want and where the volume/edition of the journal you need is located. If a journal you're after is not held in your library, you can ask the librarian to look up a list of all serials held in Australian libraries, and you can either follow it up personally or perhaps arrange an inter-library loan with the librarian.

If the library does hold the journal you want you now have to locate it on the shelf. Your library will probably use either a Library of Congress classification system or a Dewey Decimal classification system, in both of which every book has a unique identification number and items are arranged on shelves according to these numbers. Journals may be located on the main shelves with a call number amongst the books; or they may be in their own section away from the books, arranged alphabetically by title. In addition, most libraries have a special section for current serials—i.e. editions from the last 6 months or 12 months. Check with the librarian where the journals are housed. Some recent volumes may be at the bindery—ask the librarian to help you with anything you can't find. Most libraries have pamphlets on how the collection is organized and some have 'how to make the library work for you' tours. You can ask the librarian about these too.

You may not want to sit in the library to read all the articles, and you can't borrow journals, so you will probably need to photocopy some articles to read and refer to later. It's a good idea to find out first what facilities are available at the library you are going to visit (e.g. coin-operated copier, or machines which dispense copying cards for $5 notes).

Once you have collected and read the articles generated by your literature search, you will probably want to look up some of the articles mentioned in them as references. In this way your initial search has a multiplying effect. Remember, your job at this stage is to make sure you've covered the area but you still need to be discriminating. Restrict your collection to recent up-to-date articles and seminal older papers (these are the important ground-breaking articles that are cited a lot in current articles). Also look for review articles, which compare and often evaluate a number of previous research studies. Review articles can give a kick-start to the process of critically appraising the literature. We recommend that you consult *Annual Review of Public Health* which gives state of the art reviews in many useful topic areas in health promotion each year.

Critical Appraisal

What is critical appraisal?

Critical appraisal is a process of review which follows a series of questions, and which allows you to judge how useful a piece of research is for your work. Essentially you are asking:

(i) to what extent can you accept the study method and results and the conclusions drawn by the authors?

(ii) could the findings extend to other target groups, in particular your target group?

Don't be intimidated by a published article, thinking that: 'it must be good if it is in print'. Be confident in your own opinion and your own judgement about what is helpful or worthwhile and what is not.

The structure of a research article

Before going on to discuss these issues in more depth, it is important to have some idea of how research papers are structured. Research papers are generally made up of five sections: abstract; introduction; method; results; and discussion.

Abstract

An abstract is a short paragraph which summarizes what happened in the project and what was found, and gives a brief outline of theoretical and/or practical implications. Use the abstract to judge how relevant a piece of research is for your work. You may discard articles on the basis of the abstract, or you may read on. If you read on, some articles may still prove substantially different from your area of interest, but the abstract gives you a good indication.

Introduction

The introduction tells you why the authors thought that their study was worth doing and how it relates to other studies in this subject area. This section is important if you decide to include the article in your review, but initially you should read through it quickly. Come back to it later if you need details on how this paper fits into the body of research on the area.

Method

The method section tells you who the subjects were, how they were recruited, and how many there were at the beginning and end of the study. This section should also describe all the measures that were used, how they were administered, and more generally how the study was conducted (procedure). The information on subjects indicates how relevant this research is for your target group. You need to understand exactly what was actually done in the study in order to work out its validity (see below). This section is crucial to your process of critical appraisal, though, let's be frank, we can't say that this section is ever very exciting!

Results

This section tells you how the data was analysed and what results were found. These will be presented again in the context of the discussion section so again read these briefly and go back later to clarify or check points made in the discussion.

Discussion

This section presents the authors' interpretation of their findings. It also usually states any conclusions drawn, although some writers use a separate small section for conclusions. Read this section carefully, bearing in mind what the study actually did (procedure, measures, etc. from the method section) and thinking about whether the authors' claims can be justified. Sometimes authors will refer to results of other people's studies to support their own conclusions.

If you accept the authors' results and conclusions, then you must decide whether these results will apply to the group of people you are interested in. For example, will the findings from a programme run with male smokers still hold true if the programme is run with women?

When trying to decide whether to accept the findings of a study, and further, whether they apply to your own research, most of the information you need to make your decision is located in the method and results sections.

Using a summary sheet

Regardless of which question you are trying to answer, a good way to proceed is to use a separate sheet of paper for each article you read. Write the authors' names at the top of the sheet and the year of the study. On your sheet of paper make the 8 sub-headings listed below. Read through the article and attempt to write down the answers to the following questions:

1. The Research Question

What are the researchers trying to find out? Is it why people take up smoking? Is it why people can't quit if they want to? Is it how well an anti-smoking video is received by viewers? Is it how many people have given up smoking as a result of a programme? Be specific.

2. Rationale

Why is this piece of research important? What are the benefits of doing this project? The answers here follow from your description of the research question but at the 'big picture' level. Does it inform you of health needs and of barriers to change in health behaviour (needs assessment and needs analysis)? Is it part of checking the acceptability of programme materials (process evaluation)? Or is it perhaps testing whether a planned programme for improving health actually worked (impact/outcome evaluation)?

3. Study Method

How did the researchers go about their study? Was it a survey that captured a picture at one point in time (cross-sectional) or did it follow changes over time (longitudinal) by taking more than one measurement?

Did it involve one group of people; or were two or more groups compared? Were the methods used appropriate for the author's purpose?

4. Measures

What things were measured—attitudes, behaviour, social support, weight loss?

How were they measured? Did they use other people's measurement instruments or did they make up their own? If they made up their own measures, did they trial them before they used them in the study? Do you think that what they measured was appropriate?

5. Sample

How many subjects were involved in the study? Do the researchers state why they have chosen this number?

How were the study subjects selected?

Do the researchers state the number of non-respondents—was this a high number?

Who are the people to whom the study conclusions will apply?

Do you think the study subjects were representative of the larger group that the researchers were interested in?

6. Data Collection

How was the data collected (face-to-face interview, mailed questionnaire, over the phone)? Do you think this would have affected the types of results that they got? Do the authors tell you how hard they tried to get in contact with people (follow-up)?

7. Results

What results did they find? Did they report findings for particular subgroups of interest? Are any findings conflicting?

8. Discussion/Conclusions

What do the authors conclude—to what do they attribute their findings?

If a programme failed, why do they say it failed; if it was a success, why did they say it worked?

With this information in hand you have a summary of the essence of the study. In this format you can more readily assess the merits of the study, and compare the methods and results of different studies.

Fine-tuning the Literature Review to your Purpose

As mentioned earlier, whether you are looking for literature to help you with needs assessment or to help you assess a type of programme will determine which aspects of each paper you need to pay special attention to, and what additional questions you will need to ask. Most of this information you will find in the method section of the study.

There are a number of aspects you will need to consider:

- Representativeness
- Generalizability
- Appropriateness of measuring instruments
- Evaluability
- Believability
- Relative believability of conflicting findings.

Let's begin by looking at studies which you would use for understanding more about your needs assessment. In this book we encourage you to learn about your own community directly, by doing your own consultation and research with community members. You may also gain additional insights by reading about the work other people have done with similar communities.

Needs Assessment

A health survey or descriptive study describes problems or health issues within a defined group of people (this is often referred to as the study population). In order for you to be able to relate their findings to your work you must answer three broad questions as outlined below.

Representativeness—how typical were the people in the study?

The most important aspect of any descriptive study is that it should be based on a random selection or sample of the population. That is, within a specified group of people, everyone should have had an equal chance of being included in the experimental group or the control group. If the authors do not state that their sample was selected randomly, then it is less likely that their results will be typical of the general population.

Generalizability—how similar are the people in the study to your target group?

In order for other research to be useful to you, it has to be as similar as possible to your situation. That is, the people, where they live and their culture should be very similar to that of the people you are planning to study. However, it is useful to work through and answer the following questions about the group of people used in the study:

- How old were the people in the study?
- What was the proportion of men to women?
- Were people from different ethnic or language backgrounds included in the study? If they were, which ethnic/language groups were included and which were not? How might this affect the results and application of the study?
- Are the socioeconomic status and the cultural norms of the people studied different from those of the culture that you are going to study?
- Did the study group live in the city or the country?
- Were the people studied working, unemployed, or living in any special circumstances that would make them different from the group of people you are interested in studying?
- What was the setting of the research (hospital, community health centre, school)?

How appropriate were the measurement instruments used?

From your study summary page you will have a list of any instruments used to assess people's knowledge, attitudes, behaviour or health. Check whether they are common standardized instruments, or whether they were specifically developed for that research project.

Standardized instruments lend rigor to a piece of research because they have established validity and reliability, and results found by dif-

ferent researchers using the same instrument can be directly compared.
The issues of reliability and validity are:

- Can you trust that this instrument actually measures what it
  was meant to be measuring (validity)?
- Has it been shown that this instrument produces answers that
  are stable over time (test-retest reliability) and when used by
  different people (inter-observer reliability)?

If a study reports using a standard measure that you are familiar
with you probably already know its validity and reliability, and can
easily assess whether it was used appropriately in the study concerned.
If you're not familiar with the instrument, and especially if it is not
standardized (e.g. they made up their own questionnaire), you will
need to spend more time on this part of your critical appraisal. Get a
copy of the actual questions if they don't appear in the study you're
reviewing and look for evidence of reliability and validity testing in
the author's description of the methods and instruments.

Whether standardized or non-standardized, you need to be satisfied
that an instrument is reliable and valid before you can accept any findings drawn from its use. If a measurement scale does not have these
properties, then the results produced from it are unlikely to be found
again. (For more on validity and reliability of measures, see Chapter 10.

In summary, when reviewing research about descriptive studies you
need to consider whether the sample they used was representative,
whether their sample was similar to the one you are interested in
studying, and lastly whether the measurement instruments used did
measure what they were supposed to measure, and did this reliably.

Evaluating a health promotion programme—does it work?

Evaluating a health promotion programme involves some additional
steps to those outlined above. As with a descriptive study, you need to
determine the generalizability of the authors' results as well as the
reliability and validity of the measurement instruments used.

Given that the study has a representative sample, is generalizable,
and you accept that the measurement instruments used were accurate,
you now need to consider alternative explanations for the stated findings.

Evaluability—was the programme ready for its effects and results to be described? Was process evaluation carried out first?

Did the programme team check that their programme was reaching its
intended target group, being implemented the way it was planned and
that materials were appropriate and acceptable? If these steps were not
done first, it could be that the results relate to a programme that was

in effect quite different from what it was intended to be. If so, you can't judge very well whether the original idea of the programme worked or not. A lot of programmes reported in the literature leave this process out, or do not report what they did. You should be aware that this may also make programmes hard to replicate.

Believability—can you accept that the findings are a result of the programme described?

Can you believe that the changes that the authors found are a result of their programme, and not the result of something else (e.g. a television programme, or other health promotion literature sent to households at the same time); essentially, is there any alternative explanation for the findings?

Look back over the discussion of research designs presented in Chapter 6. Identify what design the authors of the paper used and think about the strengths and limitations of their study.

Relative believability—how do you decide between conflicting findings?

What happens when two different studies find conflicting results about a health promotion programme. What set of results should you believe?

Often when you have several articles in front of you, one author will conclude that the programme worked, while another will conclude that the same programme made no difference. Which authors should you believe? There are a number of things you should consider before reaching your decision:

---

1. *Did each author use a representative sample of people?*
2. *How similar were the participants (samples)? Were the participants in each study of similar age, sex, education, ethnicity, working background?*
3. *How many people dropped out of each study?*
4. *Were people who dropped out of the studies similar to the people remaining in the study?*
5. *How similar were the programmes used in each study? Were they identical? Could their slight differences account for the different findings?*
6. *Did the studies use different measurement instruments to evaluate their programmes? If yes, is this likely to have affected the results they found?*
7. *How were the programmes evaluated in each study? What study designs were used?*
8. *Were the programmes implemented properly?*

Evaluating several research articles about what appears to be the same health programme, can be a difficult task. It involves a careful look at the types of people in each study and the measurement instruments used, checking to see if any process evaluation was done and how stable the programme was before its effects were measured. Again you need to consider whether there might be alternative explanations for the results, as well as the reasons why different studies could have drawn different conclusions about the same programme, including the role of chance.

When to stop Collecting References

One of the dangers once you're on the collecting trail is to worry too much about missing that all-important article. You don't want to waste time and effort handling more literature than you need for your purpose, and you don't want to unnecessarily delay starting your programme, so you need to know when to stop. You will probably be the best judge of when you have enough information but keep in mind the following principles:

1. *It's important to review and analyse as you go. Don't just collect until you have 50 articles and then start to read. Reading as you go will also focus your attention more squarely on the immediate question and whether you've found the answer.*
2. *Don't feel obliged to read or use studies which better articles suggest are in fact irrelevant. Let the good articles (according to your critical appraisal) guide you on what to read next and what to throw out.*
3. *Stop reading and reviewing when what you've collected:*
   a) gives you a description of the issue or target group of interest in enough detail to suggest what the priority considerations might be; or
   b) provides you with enough information to design your own intervention with confidence; or
   c) bores you silly. You are training to design and evaluate better programmes. Don't let reading the literature take the spark out of you.

Summary

The essence of a good literature review is being critical about what you read and how you interpret and organize other people's ideas. It's not just a case of using what others have already done so you don't have to re-invent the wheel every time you want to go somewhere, although it's good not to have to do that! The main value in consulting the literature is that seeing the programmes and measures that have been used, and finding out what has worked and what hasn't (and therefore what hasn't been tried yet) can inspire you to be even more creative and innovative with what you use in your own setting.

Further Reading

Cooper HM. *Integrating Research: a guide for literature reviews*. Beverly Hills: Sage Publications, 1989.

Lane ND. *Techniques for Student Research: a practical guide*. Melbourne: Longman Cheshire, 1989.

Sackett DL. How to read a clinical journal. *In*: Sackett DL, Hayes RB and Tugwell P. *Clinical Epidemiology: a basic science for clinical medicine*. Boston: Little Brown and Company, 1985.

Chapter 9
HOW TO RUN A FOCUS GROUP

OBJECTIVES

At the end of this chapter you should be able to:

a) Explain what focus groups are, and when to use them.
b) Explain how to form a focus group and what factors need to be considered in the composition of focus groups.
c) Design and use a focus group interview protocol including the use of prompts and probes.
d) Explain the role of the group facilitators.
e) Analyse and collate data from groups.
f) Write a report from your focus group data.

What is a focus group?

A focus group is another name for a group interview or a group discussion, where the *focus* is on a particular topic of interest—usually a health problem or a response to a situation or issue. The group is also often focused in the sense that instead of a group of mixed people, each group focuses on people with things in common—say, people from the same ethnic group, or same age or sex, or people who are all unemployed, to name a few examples.

Focus group interviews are a relatively simple and accessible way for you to collect more information from the target group. Using a discussion outline, information is elicited from the group on a given topic or situation. The group facilitator keeps the session on track, while allowing people to talk freely and spontaneously. This draws out the range of perceptions and beliefs in the group.

The focus group is one of the methodologies used in qualitative research, when what you are principally interested in is the *range of opinion*.

A focus group interview enables you to gain a broad understanding of why participants think and act the way they do. It is not suitable for finding out how many people in your community hold a certain attitude or behave in a certain way. For example, if you wanted to find out what proportion of your target group always used condoms when they had sex, you would need to interview or give questionnaires to a representative sample of that target population instead of a focus group, but running focus groups will get you started on the *range of different attitudes* there are towards safe sex and contraception, and help you to explore the *reasons behind people's attitudes and behaviour*. Qualitative data collected from a focus group interview can provide a basis upon which to develop a questionnaire for a quantitative survey and is particularly useful in the planning stages of programme development in the health education area. Qualitative data is also important in the design and pretesting of health communications.

Guidelines for Planning Focus Groups

The success of this sort of information gathering, like most research, depends on careful planning, but all you really need to do is spend some time thinking about who it is you want to talk to, and how you're going to get them to tell you what you want to know.

Group composition

Who should be part of your group or groups?
If you are working with a small and very defined population, you could invite all of that group to participate in the focus group discussion. For example, if you are assessing the need for a postnatal follow-up service for adolescent mothers and there is only a small number of them in your area, you might be able to run one focus group with all the pregnant young women registered for delivery at the hospital that month.

In most cases, however, it would not be practical to talk to everyone from your target group. Remember that your aim is to canvass a broad range of opinion across the board, so you will need to identify the relevant subgroups within the target group and include representatives of each in your discussions. For example, if you were interested in attitudes towards condom use amongst people 25 years and under, relevant subgroups would include male heterosexuals, female heterosexuals and male homosexuals. It would probably be best to have 1 discussion group for male heterosexuals, 1 for female heterosexuals and another for male homosexuals, rather than 3 groups with a mixed membership. The reason for this is that within each subgroup of the target population, members are likely to have had similar experiences, and your focus group session can develop discussion of these experiences to a greater depth than might be possible if the groups all had participants with very different experiences. Discussion will also be freer, generally speaking, amongst groups that are relatively homogenous.

Factors to consider in regard to grouping participants include age, sex, ethnic and/or language background, education (or other indicator of socioeconomic status), employment status and area of residence. Stratifying group participants by age has also been found to be particularly important. If the discussion topic is sensitive, then it is all the more important to consider these factors as certain cultural, age and sex groupings may hinder free and open discussion.

Representativeness
As mentioned earlier, with focus groups you are interested in the range of opinion, and you will want to make sure each opinion is represented in your data. This will include opinions that are common and uncommon, strongly felt and not so strongly felt. But, unlike quantitative research, you are not interested in finding out how many of the target group hold a particular opinion, when compared with the total population. This means that you don't need to use methods such as random assignment for selecting participants and you are not trying to achieve a *representative* sample in the statistical sense.

How many people to a group?
For every focus group you should invite ten people and ideally six or seven will end up attending. This allows for refusal and non-attendance. You should begin recruiting 1 to 3 weeks in advance.

How many groups?
It is important not to over-sample from the target population. The principle is that you should continue to run focus groups until a clear pattern emerges and subsequent focus groups produce only repetitious information. That is, when the group leader starts to hear nothing new from a focus group then it is time to stop running the discussion groups and use the information from them to plan your intervention. But you won't know this in advance, so plan to run about 4 to 6 groups.

Recruitment
The usual way of locating participants for focus groups is through the informal networks of colleagues, community agencies and the target group. Sometimes you need to advertise to attract a wider range of opinions or to reach a group with low visibility in the community. Telephone calls, word of mouth and letters or talks in the community are all ways of recruiting people into your focus group discussion. When you do invite participants to attend a focus group discussion, be

sure to outline briefly what will take place and what is the purpose of the discussion.

Incentives
Because you are using people's time and experience, it may be appropriate to provide payment. This might be in the form of cash or you might offer 'payment in kind', such as movie tickets, which seems to be of more incentive than cash. However, don't preempt the situation by offering payment in advance. Many people are willing, indeed keen to participate, particularly if they preceive the benefits. Sometimes you might not be able to pay people, but your target group might still be willing to participate. To be realistic, however, some target groups, especially those which are difficult to identify and locate, will be less likely to cooperate without an incentive.

Location
The choice of location should be acceptable and convenient to focus group participants and one in which they will feel free to talk about their attitudes and opinions. For example, a baby health centre, church hall, community centre, or a hospital are all possible venues.

Designing your questions
A number of forms will need to be designed. The most important is the interview protocol, but you will also need a demographic questionnaire for participants to complete immediately prior to the focus group discussion.

The interview protocol
An interview protocol is an outline of the questions you will ask the group. Your discussion should last no longer than one and a half hours. Each question should focus on a specific issue but be broad enough to evoke a group response.

To formulate your questions you will require some basic knowledge of the target group or subject area. If you are not very familiar with the subject area then your choice of questions or areas of exploration should be based on information gleaned from preliminary talks with member of the target group, interviews with professionals working in the area and reading of the literature in this area.

The next step is to use your background understanding of the target group and the health problem or possible health problems that affect them to anticipate some of the issues. You might want to explore behavioural or environmental factors that cause the health problem. You might also want to find out about service utilization or about motivation or barriers among the target group.

Next, you need to organize these issues into a logical series of questions. Chapter 7 on questionnaire design contains some principles you should follow. The protocol may include prompts and other information to help the group facilitator achieve smooth discussion and draw people out. The first question is particularly important and should be one that is likely to include all members of the group. Try to order your questions so that you get a funnelling effect: each subsequent question narrows in further on the issues, and the discussion flows from question to answer to the next question. What you don't want is an outline that is ordered so that each new question changes the topic and breaks the flow. It's also important to leave the more sensitive questions till further along in the discussion, which tends to happen anyway if you funnel your questions.

Of course the interview protocol is only an outline. Some of the questions may not be needed by the leader—the information may be volunteered during the discussion. Similarly, flexibility must be maintained in a situation where a group opens up its own line of questioning, raising issues of importance to them which the protocol designer has not anticipated. It is often a good idea to have at least one very open question to give the group the opportunity to set or reset the agenda.

Activity
Example: Let's suppose that the rate of teenage pregnancies is higher in your town than in other similar towns in South Australia. You've decided to run a couple of focus groups to get some more information about the reasons why so many young girls are getting pregnant. Who would you have in the focus groups?

Feedback
It would be important to cover as many aspects as possible so you may run a number of focus groups with each of the following groups starting with pregnant teenagers, followed by teenage mothers, health, welfare and other workers in close contact with pregnant teenagers, parents of teenagers, and other teenagers.

Activity
What sorts of questions would you ask?

Feedback: (for the first group—teenagers now pregnant)
You anticipate that some would have become pregnant by choice, some by accident thinking they were protected against pregnancy. Others would have been aware of the risk but did not take any precautions.

Of those who did not choose to become pregnant (the majority, you anticipate), some reasons might be:

- inaccurate or lack of knowledge about sexual reproduction and contraception;
- mixed attitudes towards using contraception and/or responsibility for contraception;
- lack of self-esteem, allowing individuals to be easily influenced to have sex when unprepared;
- lack of social support, affecting decision making about contraception;
- factors such as alcohol or other drugs affecting decision making.

Putting these issues into question format, you might come out with something like the following. Always make sure, however, that there is enough freedom for you to follow up an unanticipated response.

Questions

1. *What was your first reaction when you found out you were pregnant?*
   (prompt) *Were you pleased/shocked/scared/angry?*
   (probe) *So you did/didn't want to get pregnant then?*
   (probe) *(If did) Why did you want to get pregnant?*
   (probe) *Do you still feel that way now?*

2. *Was there anyone you could tell?*
   (prompt) *Mum, Dad, friend, boyfriend, doctor, teacher?*
   (probe) *Where do you usually go if you need information or advice?*

3. *Looking back to this time last year—did you ever think you might be pregnant now? Why/Why not?*
   (prompt) *Not having sex/using the pill, condoms, etc.*
   (probe) *(if using contraception) Why do you think the pill/condom etc. didn't work?*

4. *How easy is it to say 'no' to a guy you like if you really don't want to have sex with him?*

5. *Do you think young girls should be able to say to a guy they won't have sex without a condom? How easy is it?*
   (probe) *Whose responsibility do you think it is to make sure you don't get pregnant?*
   (probe) *Do you think the guys care?*

6. *After you have the baby, would you try to get pregnant again or would you try not to get pregnant?*
   (probe) *What would you do to make sure you did't get pregnant again?*

Demographics

You will also need to design a demographic questionnaire so that you can collect basic data about your focus group participants. Your choice of questions will depend in part upon your purpose for running focus groups. You may decide to collect information about participants' age, sex, education, occupation and suburb of residence. You may like to ask some specific questions related to your area of study. For example, if you were running focus groups with migrant women you would probably want to document their country of origin and whether or not they speak English at home.

The collection of demographic information is important but not always possible. You need to find out if it is possible to collect this information from the target group (consider their literacy level) and secondly whether it is likely to alienate your group participants. For example, women from non-English-speaking backgrounds may be both reticent and unable to fill out a demographic questionnaire. In this instance you may need to note that information with the help of an interpreter or bilingual health worker. Be careful not to intimidate your participants with your information demands.

Session procedure

On arrival

It is best for one leader to run all the focus groups required for a particular health topic as this overcomes problems of reliability and also facilitates an understanding of the topic area as knowledge is accumulated. If you do need to use more than one leader then training in the background, procedure and session recording will be required. When participants arrive for the discussion, welcome them and give them a demographic questionnaire to complete.

Whether you are running one or several focus groups, it is a good idea to issue group participants with a first-name-only name tag when they arrive. The availability of refreshments before you commence the focus group(s) allows time for late arrivals and for people to fill out their questionnaire and begin to feel comfortable.

Group allocation

Most of the work of determining the composition of groups should have been done at the planning stage, but you will need to keep some flexibility to allow for non-attendance.

If you are running focus groups with all members of a target group, or with people recruited from the same club or other centre, then some participants will probably know each other. To maximize your chances of having an open discussion you can randomly allocate participants to groups on different days or groups with different facilitators. This stops peers from grouping together, which in turn frees people up to express their opinions. When working with adolescents, however, it is best to put people in groups with at least one person that they already know. So that they don't 'freeze up'.

Group facilitator

The group facilitator should be experienced in this field, able to elicit information, and at the same time prevent sidetracking and the dominance of any one member of the group. She or he should also be sensitive to cultural differences.

It is important that the group facilitator be familiar with the subject area in order to discriminate important from unimportant avenues of discussion; however she or he need not be an expert in the field. During the focus group the facilitator should not express any strong opinions about the topic area as they are likely to influence or curb the information provided by the group.

The group facilitator should emphasise that there are no right or wrong answers and should encourage the expression of different opinions and perceptions.

Leading a focus group

Group participants should be seated in a circle or semicircle or around a table. The group facilitator should organize to have shy members sit opposite with talkative members sitting beside them. Group facilitators should set the stage by introducing themselves and explaining their role and non-expert status. You will already have explained something of focus group procedure at the recruitment stage, but some aspects will need to be repeated. Time should be given here to explaining the purpose of the group, the agenda for the discussion, and the rules for the session. Rules that should be mentioned include the expectation that all members of the group will have a say, people should not speak at the same time, people should say what they think and not what they think someone else wants to hear, and that there are no right or wrong answers. Reinforce that you are interested in the range of opinions and differing points of view. Mention again the fact that you are using a tape recorder, if you are doing so.

A good way to begin the group is to let everyone introduce themselves and offer some information about themselves that relates to the purpose of the group. The group facilitator will probably want to think of a subject beforehand, such as how many children each person has, for a focus group discussion on child accidents. Then proceed to the interview protocol.

To finish, you will want to thank everyone for their participation and contribution. If you are paying participants, have the cash or ticket/voucher etc. in envelopes marked with participants' names and hand them out as you thank them.

Working with the data

Data collection

At the very minimum, data should be collected on paper, either via note taking or on butcher's paper. Using butcher's paper gives every-one in the group, not just the scribe, the opportunity to monitor what is being taken down and ensure nothing important to the group is left out. This way you are most likely to record accurately the range of opinion.

A tape recorder is recommended, especially if quotes are needed at a later date. The major drawback of using recording as the only means of data collection is that tape transcription is a very lengthy and tedious process. Taking notes as you go along is a quicker and simpler process that will give you a broad outline of the material. Later you can fill this out and illustrate points with direct quotes from the tape recording.

Whether you use a tape recorder or take notes as you go along, as soon as possible after the focus group you should write down your broad impressions, your feelings about how the group process worked and any limitations or procedural variations you were aware of. If you took notes during the focus group you should write these out in full in the next few days, expanding points as you go along. This also applies to   tape transcription. It is a good idea to write the data for each question or subject area onto a separate piece of paper. This will allow you to collate the information more easily across your focus groups.

Analysis

Qualitative data are analysed using a four-step procedure. This is a sys-tematic process and should be verifiable. That is, another person given the same data set should arrive at the same conclusions.

The steps are *organizing, shaping, summarizing,* and *explaining.* Each of these is described in turn. You will also find a discussion of qualitative data analysis in Chapter 7.

Organizing

Organizing the data means you put it in workable order. For example, if you have used butcher's paper to record the group's response you or-ganize the sheets by the order of questions, mark them clearly and then have them typed up. This gives you a more manageable way of han-dling and analysing the data. If you're used tape recordings then these will have to be transcribed in full before you can move onto the next step. At this stage you should have an overall picture of the complete data set.

Shaping

You are now ready to *shape* your data. This means you think about what patterns or themes are suggested by the data. These can relate very closely to your protocol or may be entirely different, depending on the outcome of the discussion. You need to write down the categories which seem to encompass the data and put the appropriate responses into those categories. Start with a large number of categories to indicate the broadest range of responses; in this way you are less likely to have left anything out and you will be able to answer a greater variety of questions. As you become more familiar with the material these categories can be refined and the data collapsed down as several dimensions of the one issue are located together in the same category. This leads on to the next step, summarizing.

Summarizing

When *summarizing* your data you'll be very tempted to attempt some sort of quantification of the responses. This must not happen. What you are looking for is the range or extremes of views on the nominated health topic and you do not want to know at this stage how many of those in the focus group held these views. This means that views are held by *some* and *others*, never *most* or *few*. You cannot generalize any point of view to the whole group and every view must be represented in the summary no matter if it was held by only one group member. Remember you are seeking the range of opinion held. In a subsequent population-based study you can pursue the question of how many people feel a particular way.

You should point out where the views of each group are similar and where they are dissimilar. For example, the parents of teenage parents may have said different things to the teenagers themselves.

Explaining

When you summarize your data, the central issue is one of consistency. The organizing, shaping and summarizing of your data should lead to your *explaining* of what is meant by the data.

If you feel unsure of your analysis ask a colleague to go through the process with you or do it independently. With practice you will gain more confidence and your techniques will improve. You may also decide to seek some assistance in analysing your data from an anthropologist. See Chapter 11 on finding and working with consultants.

Writing up—some guidelines

As mentioned earlier, since the members of your focus group may not be representative of the target population you should be cautious about making generalizations. It is better to restrict your discussion to the participants of your focus groups only. For example, rather than say 'General practitioners are a source of health information for women from non-English-speaking backgrounds' it would be better to say, 'In our study we found that general practitioners were a source of health information to the non-English-speaking women we interviewed'.

Again, we emphasize not to evaluate your data in quantitative terms such as percentages (i.e. x% of people said . . .). A focus group cannot give you this information. That is, nobody's opinion is systematically sought and then counted, added or subtracted. Data from focus groups are qualitative and so, as mentioned earlier, you should use words such as *some* or *others* in your report to describe your findings. This gives a general impression of the overall feeling but, more importantly, your data should tell you why these feelings were held.

When writing up your data it is useful to present and discuss it in the same order in which it was collected, that is in the order of the interview protocol. A suggested outline for writing up your data is to:

1. state the question;
2. describe the range of responses;
3. add a couple of direct quotes to illustrate the responses; and
4. provide an interpretive discussion paragraph to finish off the section.

Complete this process for each question and then provide an overall summary at the end which identifies the main themes emerging from the focus groups and any recommendations.

Further Reading

Basch CE. Focus Group Interview: An Underutilised Research Technique for Improving Theory and Practice in Health Education. *Health Education Quarterly* 1987;14(4):411–48.

Kreuger RA. Focus Group Interviews as an Evaluation Tool. An unpublished paper presented at the Evaluation Research Society and the Evaluation Network 1984 Annual Meeting, San Francisco, California.

Miles MB, Huberman AM. *Qualitative Data Analysis.* Beverly Hills: Sage Publications, 1984.

Patton MQ. *Qualitative Evaluation Methods.* Beverly Hills: Sage Publications, 1980.

US Department of Health and Human Services. *Pretesting in Health Communications. Methods, Examples and Resources for Improving Health Messages and Materials.* Public Health Service, National Institutes of Health, 1984., Chapter 2: Focus Group Interviews.

Chapter 10
WHERE TO FIND MEASURING INSTRUMENTS IN HEALTH PROMOTION

OBJECTIVES

At the end of this chapter you should be able to:

1. Explain the key attributes of standardized measures and why they are important in evaluation.
2. Define the terms 'validity' and 'reliability'.
3. Access standardized instruments which measure factors associated with health.
4. Determine the appropriateness and adequacy of available measures for a given purpose and choose the most suitable instrument.

This book includes a chapter on questionnaire design because very often you will need to design your own instruments tailored specifically to the needs of your own programme, but whenever you can it is best to use a good instrument that has been designed and tested by somebody else. This saves you the fuss. And after you have used the instrument, the data you have collected will be directly comparable to data collected by other people who have used the same instrument. This chapter is about how you go about finding measures in health promotion.

What Kinds of Measures?

First of all, as if you were designing your own instrument, you need to specify exactly what you want your measure to be able to detect. This is to make sure that it is your programme that determines the type of measure you need and not the reverse! You must clearly define which aspects of the programme you wish to evaluate. For example, you may wish to evaluate the content of the course; educators' teaching ability and interpersonal skills; participants' knowledge; attitudes and behaviour; participants' satisfaction with the course and the educator; or aspects of service delivery. You also need to be specific about the target group with whom you will be using the measure as some instruments have been designed specifically for some groups. For example, for measuring social support, Barrera has designed an instrument specifically for use with pregnant adolescents.[1] Henderson and his colleagues have developed a social support instrument for use with the elderly.[2]

The chapter on impact and outcome evaluation indicated some of the different types of factors you might want to measure with your health promotion programme. Specific instruments have been developed for a range of different types of factors that may be the focus of your health promotion programme and a sample of these is indicated in the following table.

Location of Measures

Writing to authors: the direct approach
Part of the task when you are reading the literature is to observe how the authors measured the factors of interest. Often you will find the questions they asked of their target group or programme participants reproduced in the table of results. If authors talk about a questionnaire they have developed for a study you may find a footnote saying that copies of the questionnaire are available by writing to one of the authors and the address is given. When you do take an opportunity to correspond, it is always good practice to let the author know how you will be using their measure and volunteer to inform them how your study goes. You should also assure them that you will acknowledge their part in developing the instrument. Writing to authors can also be very rewarding as they may also send you more details about their work and helpful references.

Instrument banks
There are a number of places where testing resources are held that you might want to go to shop for an instrument. For example, you can get a copy of a psychological measure from the Australian Psychological Society. Since most of these resource centres are run by professional associations, there are often some restrictions on their access and/or use by people who are not members of the appropriate profession. See the psychologist at your community health centre or hospital for advice.

Table 13. *Some measures for use in health promotion.*

Name of Measure	Use	Authors
1. Health Locus of Control	Measures extent to which a person feels their health status is determined by their own actions or by forces external to them	Wallston & Wallston[3]
2. Beck Depression Inventory	Measures depth of depression; uses self-reporting	Beck et al[4]
3. Patient Satisfaction	Measures people's satisfaction with aspects of care such as accessibility, efficacy and technical quality	Ware et al[5]
4. Caregiver Quality of Life Index (CQLI)	Carogivers value their current quality of life against alternative scenarios which is used as a measure of the effect of prolonged caregiving on the respondents health	Mohide et al[6]
5. Coping Health Inventory for Parents (CHIP)	Assesses the extent to which parents are coping with a child's chronic illness	McCubbin et al[7]
6. Activities of Daily Living Scales (ADL)	Measure the extent to which people (usually the elderly or disabled) are able to perform independently routine self-care tasks such as dressing, bathing, etc.	Katz et al[8]
7. Instrumental Activities of Daily Living Scales (IADL)	Similar to above but includes other functions such as shopping, using the telephone, etc.	Lawton[9]
8. Sickness Impact Profile (SIP)	Similar to ADL; the SIP gives behavioural measures of dysfunction in physical and psychosocial dimensions and in general life management	Bergner et al[10]
9. Adult Patterns of Tobacco Use in Australia	Measures respondent's attitudes toward smoking and health-related issues as well as prevalence of smoking in adult populations	Hill and Gray[11]
10. Tobacco and Alcohol Use among Australian secondary school children	Measures prevalence of and alcohol use in secondary school children	Hill et al[12]

Table 13. — *continued*

Name of Measure	Use	Authors
11. Ward Atmosphere Sale	Measures the social environment created by staff and patients in a treatment setting, e.g., staff control, patient involvement, personal problem orientation	Moos[13]
12. Community-oriented Programmes Environment Scale	Similar to above but adapted for halfway houses, day treatment programs, etc.	Moos et al[14]
13. Group Environment Scale	Measures the social climate created by a group of people (say a self-help group, a working group, etc.). Measures aspects such as cohesion, order and organization, leader support, etc.	Moos et al[15]
14. Social Support Availability and Adequacy (abbreviated version of the Interview Schedule for Social Interaction)	Measures: (1) the number of fairly close social ties a person has, including confidants, partner; and (2) how adequate the person feels this level of support is	Henderson et al[2]
15. Social Support in the adjustment of pregnant adolescents	Similar to above but specific to and validated for pregnant adolescent respondents	Barrera[1]
16. National Heart Foundation Risk Factor Survey (has section on food frequency)	Measures how often food items on a comprehensive list of foods are consumed and the amounts eaten	National Heart Foundation[16]
17. Life Events Scale (for heterosexual respondents)	Measures the number of critical events (such as marriage, changing jobs, moving house) and measures how much stress the respondent feels from these events (Australian and New Zealand)	Tennant and Andrews[17,18]
18. Gay Life events scale for homesexual men (GALES)	As above, but has been normed in Australian conditions for homosexual men	Rosser and Ross[19]
19. Homosexual attitudes to condom use scale (HATC)	Measures attitudinal factors concerning condom use as a prophylaxis for AIDS. Validated for male homosexual populations (Australian)	Ross[20]

Table 13. — *continued*

Name of Measure	Use	Authors
20. General Health Questionnaire	Measures not general but mental health, in particular mental impairment other than psychosis.	Goldberg[21]
21. Malaise Inventory	Measures psychosomatic symptoms associated with emotional distress. Useful for assessing carer malaise.	Rutter et al[22]

Professional networks

Most of the instruments we have listed are widely used already and are appropriate for a broad range of programmes, but there is also a growing need for measures of new areas of interest and for specific populations. There may be really good instruments that are not yet widely available, but have been validated and are now being used by graduate students, academics and other people involved in developing standard measures. If you can develop or use existing networks that link you with research departments in hospitals or universities in this way, you will get to know what new advances are being made and some might be useful for evaluating your programmes. And you might be surprised by a spin off from collaborative research between academics (theory) and your (practical) programme application. Again, the only caution is to make sure you select an appropriate measure.

How Do You Know That it is a Good Measure?

In choosing which measure you are going to use, the following questions will help you assess the quality of other people's instruments and how appropriate they might be for your purpose.

Look for discussion of the purpose of the instrument and the concepts it aims to measure and discussion of populations for which the instrument is appropriate. To do this you might need to seek out articles published separately from the instrument itself, which describe how each instrument was developed and used. These articles can also provide helpful hints on difficulties, hints on analysis or modifications of the instrument.

Instruments that have been used before usually have established validity and reliability. That is, someone has demonstrated that the questionnaire they have developed to measure symptoms, for example, is really measuring symptoms and not how the person feels about their health (validity) and that if a respondent were to fill out a questionnaire twice, with several intervening weeks or months, they would answer those same questions almost identically on both occasions (reliability), provided of course that there had been no real change in their condition. In effect you need to ask whether you can trust that each instrument is measuring what it is meant to be measuring, and whether it produces answers that are stable over time.

Validity

1. *Does the instrument really measure what it sets out to measure? Have its results been shown to compare well with other established measures - e.g. does the number of cigarettes people say they smoke on a questionnaire compare well with cotinine levels measured in their saliva?*

Reliability

2. *Has it been shown that you get the same results with this instrument when used on different occasions (test-retest reliability) in the absence of real change?*
3. *Has it been shown that you get the same results with this instrument when it is used by different people (inter-observer reliability)?*

Some examples might help here. The question 'What is your birth-date?' is usually answered reliably. That is, regardless of when you ask it or how long it is since you last asked it people will give you the same answer. In contrast, the question 'On how many occasions in the last 10 years have you been taking the contraceptive pill for periods longer than 12 months?' will probably not be answered reliably. However, in trying to get accurate information from people over a range of topics researchers have developed different questioning techniques which improve the reliability of responses. This is why different instruments or questionnaires trying to measure the same thing may have different reliabilities—because of how the question is framed.

The next set of questions requires you to think more about the instrument in terms of what you want it to do in relation to your own study or evaluation.

In summary then, trying to find a measurement instrument for use in your own study requires that you define which aspects of your programme you are going to measure. You then have to find an instrument that looks appropriate for your setting, that is used with target groups similar to yours, that is not too long, is administered the way you want, and that gives valid and reliable answers. Once you've done this thoroughly you can be confident of the measurements you make and of using them in evaluation.

Comprehensiveness of measurement scale

4. Does the measurement scale under consideration measure all the aspects of the programme you are interested in assessing? For example, if you want to measure people's social support, does the measure include support at work as well as outside the work environment?

Sensitivity

5. Will the instrument to able to register the sort of changes you are hoping to detect? For example, if you want to measure improvements in the quality of life of patients with end-stage cancer, will the instrument register small changes at the end of the spectrum of quality of life?

Reasonableness

6. Does the instrument you are considering look like a reasonable instrument to you? (i.e. if you were asked to fill it out as a programme participant would you be able to do so with ease; would you see it as relevant?)

7. As a participant of the programme you wish to evaluate would you be able to understand the questions asked, or are some of the words and concepts used too difficult? Take into account the age and/or educational level of the people in your programme.

8. How long is the instrument? Will the length of the instrument deter people from filling it out accurately?

Data type

9. What types of responses is the participant required to give? Are questions open ended or can a given answer be circled? (Use open-ended if you want qualitative data, otherwise answers that can be ticked or circled.) Will the responses collected provide you with too little or too much detail?

Administration and scoring

10. How is the instrument administered? Do you have to interview participants or can they fill it in themselves?
11. How do you score the instrument?

References

1. Barrera MJ. Social support in the adjustment of pregnant adolescents. *In* Gottlieb BH (ed). *Social Networks and Social Support.* Beverley Hills: Sage Publications, 1981.

2. Henderson AS, Duncan-Jones P, Byrne DG. Availability and Adequacy of Social Support (shortened for of the Interview Schedule for Social Interaction). *Neurosis and the Social Environment.* Academic Press Australia, 1981.

3. Wallston KA, Wallston BS. Health locus of control scales. *Research in the Locus of Control Contruct Vol 1: Assessment Methods.* New York: Academic Press, 1981.

4. Beck AT, Ward CH, Mendelson M, Mock J, Erbaugh J. An Inventory for Measuring Depression. *Archives of General Psychiatry* 1961;4:53–63.

5. Ware JE, Davies-Avery A, Stewart AL. The measurement and meaning of patient satisfaction. *Health and Medical Care Services Review* 1978;1:1–22.

6. Mohide AE, Torrance GW., Streiner DL, Pringle DM, Gilbert R. Measuring the wellbeing of family caregivers using the time trade-off techique. *Journal Clinical Epidemiology* 1988;5:475–482.

7. McCubbin MA, Patterson JM, Cauble AE, Wilson LR, Warwick W. CHIP— Coping Health Inventory for Parents: An assessment of parental coping patterns in the care of the chronically ill child. *Journal of Marriage and Family* 1983;45:359–370.

8. Katz S, Ford AB, Moskowitz RW, Jackson BA, Jaffee MW. Studies of Illness in the Aged. The Index of ADL: A Standardized measure of Biological and Psychological Function. *Journal of the American Medical Association* 1963; 185:94ff.

9. Lawton MP. The functional assessment of elderly people. *Journal of American Geriatrics Society* 1971;19:645–681.

10. Bergner M, Bobbitt RA, Carter W, Gilson BS. The Sickness Impact Profile: Development and final revision of a Health Status Measure. *Medical Care* 1981;19:787–805.

11. Hill D, Gray N. *Adult Population Smoking Prevalance Survey.* Available from the Centre for Behavioural Research in Cancer. Anti-Cancer Council of Victoria. 1 Rathdowne Street, Carlton South Vic.3053.

12. Hill D. Willcox S, Gardner G, Houston J. *Cigarette and Alcohol Consumption among Australian Secondary Schoolchildren in 1984.* Available from the Centre for Behavioural Research in Cancer Anti-Cancer Council of Victoria, 1 Rathdowne Street, Carlton South Vic.3053.

13. Moos RH. *Evaluating Treatment Environments: A Social Ecological Approach.* New York: John Wiley and Sons, 1974.

14. Moos RH, Grauvain M, Max SW, Mehren B. Assessing the environments of sheltered care settings. *The Gerontologist* 1979;19:74–82.

15. Moos RH, Insel PM, Humphrey B. *Preliminary Manual for family environment scale, work environment scale and group environment scale.* Palo Alto, California: Consulting Psychologists Press, 1974.

16. National Heart Foundation. *Risk Factor Survey.* Available from the National Heart Foundation, 343 Riley Street, Surrey Hills NSW 2010, or your state office.

17. Tennant C, Andrews G. A scale to measure the stress of life events. *Australian and New Zealand Journal of Psychiatry* 1976;10:27–32.

18. Tennant C, Andrews G. A scale to measure the cause of life events. *Australian and New Zealand Journal of Psychiatry* 1977;11:163–167.

19. Rosser BS, Ross MW. A Gay Life Events Scale for Homosexual Men (GALES). *Journal of Gay and Lesbian Pschotherapy* 1988;1:2.

20. Ross MW. Attitudes toward condoms as AIDS prophylaxis in homosexual men: dimensions and measurement. *Psychology & Health* 1988;2:291–299.

21. Goldberg DP. *The Detection of Psychiatric Illness By Questionnaire*. London: Oxford University Press, 1972.

22. Rutter M, Tizard J, Whitmore K. *The Malaise Inventory in Education health and behaviour*. London: Longmans, 1970.

Further Reading

Donald CA, Ware JE Jr, Brook RH, Avery AD. Conceptualization and Measurement of Health for Adults in the Health Insurance Study, vol. IV. *Social Health*, (R-1987/4-HEW). Santa Monica, Calif.: Rand Corporation, 1978.

Duke University Center for the Study of Aging and Human Development. *Multidimensional Functional Assessment: The OARS Methodology*. Durham NC: Duke University, 1978.

Ewan C. *Teaching skills development manual—a guide for teachers of health workers*. Sydney: University NSW, 1984.

Gilson BS, Gilson JS, Bergner M, Bobbitt RA, Kressel S, Pollard WE, Vesselago M. The Sickness Impact Profile. Development of an Outcome Measure of Health Care. *American Journal of Public Health* 1975;65:1304–1310.

Good MJD, Smilkstein G, Good BJ, Shaffer T, Arons T. The Family APGAR Index: A Study of Construct Validity. *Journal of Family Practice* 1979;8:557–582.

Graney MJ, Graney EE. Scaling Adjustment in Older People. *International Journal on Aging and Human Development* 1973;4:351–359.

Graney MJ, Graney EE. Communications Activity Substitutions in Aging. *Journal of Communication* 1974;24:88–96.

Gurland B, Kuriansky J, Sharpe L, Simon R, Stiller P, Birkett P. The Comprehensive Assessment and Referral Evaluation (CARE)—Rationale, Development and Reliability: Part II. A factor analysis. *International Journal of Aging and Human Development* 1977;8:9–42.

Hall J, Masters G. Measuring outcomes of health services: a review of some available measures. *Community Health Studies* 1986;10:147–155.

Katz S, Hedrick S, Henderson N. The Measurement of Long-Term Care Needs and Impact. *Health and Medical Care Services Review* 1979;2:2–21.

Marsh H.W. Students' evaluations of university teaching: dimensionnality, reliability, validity, potential biases and utility. *Journal of Educational Psychology* 1984; 76(5):707–754.

Melzack R. The McGill Pain Questionnaire: Major Properties and Scoring Methods. *Pain* 1975;1:227–299.

Morris LL, Fitz-Gibbon CT. *How to measure achievement*. Beverly Hills: Sage Publications, 1978.

Peterson WA, Mangen DJ, Sanderrs R. *The Development of an Instrument Bank: Assessment of Available Instruments and Measurement Scales for the Study of Aging and the Elderly: Final Report*. Kansas City, Mo.: Midwest Council for Social Research in Aging, 1978.

Sidle A, Moos R, Cady P, Adams S. Development of a Coping Scale. *Archives of General Psychiatry* 1969;20:226–232.

Ware JE Jr, Johnston SA, Davies-Avery A, Brook RH. Conceptualization and Measurement of Health Status for Adults in the Health Insurance Study, col. III *Mental Health* R-1987/3-HEW. Santa Monica, Calif.: Rand Corporation, 1979.

Chapter 11
GETTING HELP: FINDING AND WORKING WITH CONSULTANTS

OBJECTIVES

At the end of this chapter you should be able to:

1. Identify the types of consultants that may be useful to you in programme evaluation.
2. Locate these consultants for your own area or region.
3. Work out a relationship between yourself and the consultant which is satisfying to both parties.

This book is intended to be a do-it-yourself guide in health promotion evaluation but do-it-yourself does not have to mean doing it on your own. This chapter is about the sort of people you can call on to help you with programme evaluation. We will focus on what they can offer, your joint expectations and how to work together so that both parties find satisfaction. On many occasions you probably also act as a consultant to other people so it is good to examine the situation from both points of view.

What is a consultant? A consultant is simply someone you go to for expert advice. Often this is a colleague and the interaction is quite informal, but on many occasions you may make an appointment to go and see someone specially and this creates a slightly different situation with possibly different expectations.

Why Might You Need to Use Consultants?

There may be many occasions along the pathway from needs assessment to outcome evaluation when you might need the advice and assistance of someone with more skill or expertise. There is no shame in this! Statistics, for example, is an area where most of us need help! A consultant is simply a person who has chosen to be involved exclusively in areas which you may only touch on occasionally. It makes sense to use the skills of others to complement your own.

Activity
Can you list the sorts of occasions in programme development and evaluation when you might need the help of a consultant? What sort of tasks might you hope they could help you with?

Feedback
The following might give you an indication of the sort of occasions on which it is common for some people to seek help, though each person's list will differ according their own needs:

- analysis and interpretation of health status and census data
- questionnaire design
- choice of measurement instruments
- choosing a sample and sample size
- statistical analysis
- qualitative data analysis
- interpretation and presentation of results
- study design in impact and outcome evaluation
- costing.

When is the best time to approach a consultant? The answer is early in the planning of the approach you will take and NOT so late that what you really require is 'rescuing'. It is also better if you have spent some time thinking carefully about the problem, the rationale behind the approach you are taking and the alternatives you think may be open to you before you see the consultant. This will simply assist in communication. If your programme and your problem are not well articulated, your consultant will find it hard to work out exactly how they can help you. Both parties will be frustrated. The other thing to remember is that all consultation does not have to be problem oriented. It is always helpful to set up occasions where you present your work to colleagues and others for discussion. This may generate ideas which may strengthen your project.

Types of Consultants and Where to Find Them

The following list is not exhaustive, but should cover the main sorts of people you might like to seek out. Remember, however, that regardless of their discipline or training individuals will vary in their aptitude, interests and experience.

Statisticians

Let's say that you have done a survey in your area and found that of the 120 people in your sample, 57 (47.5%) are smokers. Is this likely to be an accurate estimate of the true proportion of smokers in your community? Does it really indicate that smoking in your community is a priority health problem (given that your figure is above the Australian population average of 33%)?

Let's consider another example. You have conducted a smoking cessation programme and have found that at the end of the programme 25% of people have quit smoking compared to 19% of people on the waiting list ready to go into the next programme. Can you conclude that your programme is a success?

These are the sorts of problems that you should consult a statistician about. Their training is in mathematics, especially probability theory, and its application to statistical data analysis. A statistician will be able to advise you on many aspects of study design and research methods which are important for ensuring that the conclusions of your study will be valid. So before you set out to collect your data you can talk to a statistician about sample selection, sample size, study design and formatting a questionnaire to make it easier for analysis. A statistician can also advise on methods of data analysis and interpretation and presentation of results.

Few community health services employ statisticians specifically for the purpose of advising on health research design. People with these sort of skills are often completely engaged by health departments in the collation, analysis and interpretation of large health data sets and databases. Increasingly, however, statisticians who may be able to assist you in some of these areas are being employed (on a part-time basis) in the clinical departments of major hospitals to support their research programmes. So this may be an access point for some health workers. University departments of public health, community health, health administration, health sciences and community medicine nearly always have a full-time statistician on staff. At some universities the statistics department offers a consulting service to the public. This is also true for other major tertiary institutions. Statisticians with a particular interest in the applications of their field in the health arena are often members of the Biometric Society and you can access this group by making enquiries at the Australian Institute of Health in Canberra. This may be of particular help to health workers in rural regions who could enquire about the people in their own area.

Epidemiologists

Epidemiologists are interested in the distribution of health and disease in populations and the extent to which these patterns can be explained by a range of factors: behavioural, social, physiological, genetic, environmental, economic and so on. This study attempts to elucidate the causal pathways contributing to illness and health and thereby pinpoint factors for intervention. Increasingly, epidemiologists have also been involved in the evaluation of the interventions that have been designed to address some of these factors.

Training in epidemiology is undertaken at a postgraduate level. The undergraduate training of epidemiologists is usually either in medicine, statistics or the behavioural and social sciences.

You can consult an epidemiologist about sources of health data, sample selection, questionnaire design, and study design. An epidemiologist may also know something about the factors which you wish to study in relation to your health problem, and what is known about the methods of measurement of these factors. This can be a highly specialized area, so some epidemiologists may be good on the measurement of dietary fat while others may be better advisors in the area of measurement of alcohol intake or smoking. They may also have up-to-date information about research projects and evaluations in your field of interest.

Epidemiologists can be found in university and hospital departments of public health, community health, epidemiology, community medicine, health services research and health administration. Many health departments also have epidemiology and prevention units where you can seek advice and support for your projects. Some of the Commonwealth and state organizations involved in health (for example, the National Heart Foundation, the Anti-Cancer Council of Victoria) also employ epidemiologists in their research units. You can also consult a list of members of the Australian Epidemiological Association (AEA), who can be contacted via the Australian Institute of Health in Canberra. Many epidemiologists are also members of the Public Health Association, whose contact address is listed at the back of the book.

Behavioural and Social Scientists

People trained in the various branches of psychology and in sociology, social work and anthropology can assist with a range of issues. The training of most psychologists, for example, includes a hefty component in research design and statistical analysis. They are also particularly useful in advising you about the state of the art in relation to many measures of individual and social fuctioning (such as locus of control, self-esteem, social support, and so on). Similarly, social workers and sociologists may have had experience with the sort of measures you may wish to select for use in your evaluation. A great deal of social research is conducted using survey methodologies, so social scientists are particularly good for advice about questionnaire design, wording of sensitive questions, how to boost response rates, training of interviewers and so on.

Health and health promotion research in recent years seems to have been undergoing a 'rediscovery' of qualitative methods in health problem investigation and also in evaluation. This is the sort of technique that anthropologists, in particular, have been using for years. Asking a lot of open-ended questions might seem quite straightforward, but it is easy to misuse this technique. Analysing data from qualitative investigations can also be quite daunting without some advice on some relatively simple and efficient approaches. It also may be useful to consult an anthropologist at the beginning of your study to get advice on the sort of methods you might use to observe and learn about your target group, particularly if you are working outside your own cultural group.

However, many aspects of the social sciences have become highly specialized, which makes it a little difficult for 'outsiders' (or even 'insiders') to shop for consultants. Within psychology, for example, many health psychologists have a behavioural approach and are best for advising on lifestyle programmes with a focus on individual behaviour change. Community psychologists on the other hand could advise on measures to use in the evaluation of community development programmes. They are likely to suggest measures that focus on changes occurring on levels other than the individual (social environment, community competence and so on). Both sociology and anthropology have within them sub-disciplines of medical sociology and medical anthropology which are likely to overlap more with your interests than the mainstream of each discipline.

Where do you find these people? Fortunately, many of these consultants are getting a little closer to home. As well as in all the public health type departments listed earlier, you can look for them in departments of social work, sociology, psychology and anthropology in universities and major tertiary institutions. Many people skilled in these areas are employed as research officers in health and community service departments and in some states they are in community health centres. Again we suggest you seek out membership listings from associations that are trying to develop and foster networks in this area. These include the Public Health Association of Australia (PHA), the Community Health Association and the Australasian Evaluation Society. Some useful addresses are at the back of this book.

Health Economists

Health economists are a special breed of economists whose area of interest is efficiency, equity, organization and financing of health services and health care interventions. The terminology of cost effectiveness and cost–benefit analysis is frequently misused by other groups within the health services, so a health economist will clarify this for you and help you to perhaps re-educate the health care administrators who demand this type of evidence.

Other areas which are frequently misunderstood are how to cost health care services, taking into consideration, for example, marginal costs, rather than simply average costs and also 'discounting' costs over time. The complexity of this area, and the frequency with which the novice makes mistakes, makes it imperative that you consult a health economist. Because assessments of costs often go side by side with assessments of effects, many health economists have also specialized in the measurement and 'scoring' of health outcomes, such as quality of life and 'quality adjusted life years'. You may find that they can be of help to you in these areas also.

Health economics is a relatively new field and there are not many health economists around. The first enquiry point should be in the university and hospital public health type departments mentioned earlier. Health service research units in health departments may also employ these people. Many health economists are members of the Health Economists Group and again this group can be contacted by first enquiring at the Australian Institute of Health.

Working with consultants

The satisfaction of both parties will depend to a large extent on how well you first negotiate the consultant's role. What are they to get out of it? How often will you expect to see them? What sort of responsibilities do you wish to share? What responsibilities do you wish to split between you? Is the role simply an advisory one or do you want the consultant to work on the project and take on some major tasks? Is this simply a 'one-off' or do you hope to set up an ongoing relationship?

Payments, publications and agreements

The consultant may be working within a health department where their duty statement includes providing a service to people like you. This situation is very different from that where the consultant is an academic or where the consultant is in private practice. Are you offering payment to the consultant or are the rewards intangible? Most people will offer some initial advice free and without obligation from either side. After that there needs to be some reward for the investment of the consultant's time. If this is to be money, then the basis for this must be clear. But there are many rewards and motives for working in this area that are not financial. If your consultant is a statistician, you may find even if they make no charges for their services you may be expected to pay for data entry costs and computer time. These types of costs, however, are only incurred in larger studies.

Many consultants will be interested in maintaining the quality of the evaluation research you are undertaking to a publishable standard. This is particularly true for academics whose promotion prospects depend heavily on their publications. Whether or not these consultants request payment (and many don't), reward for them will come in writing a paper. Authorship of this paper should be discussed early, to prevent any subsequent misunderstandings or bad feelings, particularly about who will be the senior (first) author on the paper. A common happy compromise is where the consultant and programme designer write up two papers: one with a programme focus, where the programme designer takes first author, and one with a research focus, where the consultant takes first author. Another practice is to separate responsibility for the reporting of the process evaluation from the reporting of the impact or outcome evaluation.

Consultants in private practice have to make a living from their work and frequently they can only commit themselves to major or substantial projects. They also may be interested in publications, but usually less so than academics.

Some of the major funding organizations in health promotion will support groups and agencies to engage an evaluation consultant to take over the primary responsibility for the evaluation component of the project they have funded. Often you are encouraged to commit the consultant to a formal agreement regarding the nature of the service they are expected to provide and the conditions associated with this. A contract which both parties sign covers such aspects as reporting, copyright of material produced by the consultant as part of the project, disclosure of information to third parties, payment procedures, indemnity for accidents occurring on the job, procedures for the handling of disputes and procedures for the handling of conflicts of interest.

Communication

As we mentioned earlier, the quality of the interaction with your consultant will depend greatly on how well you can describe your project and the issues it presents. It is very important to fill them in, even on the areas which may not seem directly relevant, as this gives the consultant a perspective on the project and where their contribution fits in.

After the consultant has given you some time and advice, it is also courteous to keep them informed of your progress. You must ask before you put the consultant's name on any reports or submissions. This is particularly important in case funding bodies contact them independently. You won't do the project any good if the consultant is put on the spot answering questions about a project they can hardly remember!

Although we expect you to choose your consultant on the basis of their knowledge and skills and not their personality, it is important that they be the sort of person with whom you can discuss things freely. You both need to create a positive climate between you that allows close scrutiny of your project and their contribution without defensiveness. Giving and receiving criticism constructively is a skill and not all consultants and consultees work on it sufficiently.

It is important to keep a record of the decisions and suggestions covered in your conversations with your consultant. We are not recommending that you keep formal minutes, but it might be a good idea to write to a consultant on occasions, just listing what you understand the outcomes of your discussions to have been. This is a good way of making sure that both parties keep track of what is going on.

Role delineation and expectations

We may have created the impression that the consultant should be treated as some kind of oracle, or special being. Remember that it is your project and it exists as a result of your initiatives, talent and skills. Don't lose this perspective. You should work out with the consultant exactly what their role will be. This can be advisor, supervisor, joint investigator, sounding board or someone who undertakes special tasks (e.g., statistical analysis). Of course, the consultant's role may also change across time depending on the demands of the project.

Remember that your consultant may be a specialist in a narrow field and they are unlikely to have had the benefit of the sort of experience and training you have received in health promotion programme development and practice. Particularly to some consultants with a strong background in experimental evaluation research, the notion of process evaluation and evaluability assessment may be foreign. Indeed, many of the premature and inappropriate evaluations that have occurred in the past have been directed by people with little understanding of what was in the 'black box' called the programme.[1] It may be up to you to provide this perspective. Do it with confidence!

References

1. Smith NL. The feasibility and desirability of experimental methods in evaluation. *Evaluation and Program Planning* 1980;(3):251–256.

Further Reading

Dobson A, Hall J. Uses and Abuses of consultants. *Transactions of the Menzies Foundation. A Handbook for Researchers.* 1984;7:81–84.

Glossary

Activities Products, services or resources offered to programme participants as part of a health promotion programme, e.g. a small-group education session on over-the counter medications.

At risk Describes an individual or group that is considered more susceptible to a certain health problem than the rest of the population, by virtue of their biological, social or economic status, behaviour or environment (*contributing factors/risk factors*; see also *risk marker*).

For example, people who smoke are at a high risk of contracting lung cancer.

The increased susceptibility of an individual or a group to a health problem can be quantified relative to the general population. This is known as relative risk.

Attitude—see **health attitude**

Behaviour—see **health behaviour**

Behavioural epidemiology The study of the distribution and prevalence of behavioural determinants of disease and ill health.

Community In modern societies, especially highly urban societies, individuals rarely belong to a single distinct community but maintain membership of a range of communities based on variables such as geography, occupation, social contact, values, leisure interests and other important features of their lives; e.g. gay community, hearing and non-hearing communities, Christian community, academic community.

Community development Refers to the process of facilitating the community's awareness of the factors and forces which affect their health and quality of life, and ultimately helping to empower them with the skills needed for taking control over and improving those conditions in their community which affect their health and way of life. It often involves helping them to identify issues of concern and facilitating their efforts to bring about change in these areas.

Community organization Linking community groups and structures and residents together over common issues and helping to facilitate organizational efforts to bring about change.

Community participation (community involvement) Involving people in the processes which affect their health. Some people use this term to refer to involving people in health promotion activities. Others use it to refer to involvement in decision-making structures that affect health, including intersectoral approaches to community health planning and promotion. Most effective participation occurs when a community's skills have been developed (community development), that is, when a community is skilled in the processes of participation and decision making.

Contributing factor   Any aspect of behaviour, society, or the environment, or anything else which contributes to a *risk factor* for a *health problem*, e.g. not having easy access to purchase condoms is a contributing factor for having sex without a condom, which is in turn a risk factor for contracting HIV.

Contributing factors *predispose, enable* or *reinforce* risk factors, which are linked directly with the health problem. (See entries for *predisposing, enabling* and *reinforcing* factors).

Some authors distinguish between risk factors and contributing factors on the basis that one is causally linked and the other is not but we prefer to maintain a distinction on the basis that a risk factor is directly linked with the health problem and a *contributing factor* is linked to the health problem via the risk factor—that is, it is a factor which contributes to or helps to explain the risk factor.

Comparison group   A group of people with similar characteristics to the participants in a health programme, but who do not receive the programme. The two groups are compared over time, as a measure of programme effects. (See also *control group, programme group, experimental group, equivalent groups, non-equivalent groups.*)

Control group   A type of comparison group, where the people are allocated to the experimental group or the comparison group at random. That is, the two groups are drawn randomly from the same population. (See also *equivalent groups, randomized controlled trial*; compare with *non-equivalent groups; quasi-experimental.*)

Decision makers   People who make decisions about the allocation of resources for existing and future programmes; those people to whom reports evaluating health programmes are usually submitted, e.g. health administrators; representatives of government or funding bodies.

Effectiveness   The ability of an intervention to achieve its intended effect in those to whom it is offered; that is, its ability in practice or effect in the real world (after Last). Effectiveness concerns the question 'Does it work?'

For example, when measuring the effectiveness of legislation aimed at preventing the spread of legionnaire's disease, researchers take into account the effect of an estimated level of non-compliance with the legislation.

Efficacy   The ability of an intervention to achieve its intended effect in those individuals who comply under optimal conditions; effect in an ideal world. Efficacy concerns the question 'Can it work?'

For example, when measuring the efficacy of legislation aimed at preventing the spread of legionnaire's disease, researchers assume that the public will comply with the rules set down.

Efficiency   The effectiveness of a programme (improvement in health) in relation to costs (in terms of time, labour, material consumed). Participant discomfort or other costs may be taken into account (after Last).

Note: Sometimes used to refer only to costs, without considering outcome.

Enabling factor   Any characteristic of an individual, group or the environment that facilitates health behaviour or other conditions affecting health, including any skill or resource required to attain that condition (after Green). Enabling factors can facilitate conditions that lead to ill health or conditions that lead to good health.

For example, lack of easy access to contraceptives; availability of healthy takeaway food.

Epidemiology   The study of the distribution and determinants of health-related states and events in human populations (after Last). Traditionally this study has been applied to the control of disease, but it is now increasingly applied to disease prevention and health promotion. (See also *behavioural epidemiology* and *social epidemiology*.)

Equivalent groups design   An experimental design where members are allocated to the experimental group and the control group by *random assignment*, that is, members have an equal chance of being allocated to the experimental group or the control group. The purpose of this is to produce two groups with an even distribution of factors which may influence outcome.

Evaluable   Able to be fairly or appropriately judged or evaluated; a programme is evaluable when its activities, goals and objectives are articulated in such a way as to provide meaningful and measurable information for the evaluator to present to the decision-maker. The programme is also being implemented appropriately. (See *evaluability assessment*.)

Evaluability assessment   Prepares the way for impact and outcome evaluation by:

1.   checking that the programme is able and ready to be evaluated and making any adjustments necessary;

2.   ensuring that the structure of the evaluation (questions asked, terms of reference etc.) will provide sufficient relevant information to those who make the final decision about the programme's worth;

3   identifying *users* for the evaluation and the information they want (they are usually *decision makers* but also include staff and consumer groups).

While most of these aspects should have been addressed during the needs assessment, programme planning or process evaluation stages, the evaluability assessment acts as a failsafe mechanism to ensure that the time and effort spent in full-scale impact and outcome evaluation is not wasted.

Evaluation   The process by which we decide the worth or value of something (Suchman). For health promotion, this process involves measurement and observation (*evaluation research*) and comparison with some criterion or standard (usually a programme goal).

Evaluation research   Observations and measurements (research) made for the purpose of evaluation.

Experimental group   A group of people involved in an experiment who receive an intervention, as compared with the *comparison group*, who receive no intervention.

For example, an experimental group of diabetics take part in a nutrition education programme; control group diabetics do not take part in the programme, to assess programme effects. The experimental group equates with the programme group or intervention group in terms of programme planning. Allocation into groups is ideally by random assignment.

Formative evaluation Evaluation for the purpose of improving the programme as it is being implemented.

Goal (programme goal; health goal) The desired long-term outcome of a health intervention; such as a reduction in the health problem or improvement in health status. It is measureable (how much improvement, by when, by whom). E.g. to reduce death rate from cancer of the cervix by 30% by the year 2000.

In some literature, such as *Health for All Australians*, *target* is used to refer to time-specific and measureable desired changes; while *goals* refer to broad aspirations which do not specify time frames or degrees of change (in this case the goal would be to reduce the incidence of death from cancer of the cervix; the target would be to reduce the incidence of death from cancer of the cervix by 30% by the year 2000). Still other literature refers the concept of measureable and time-spacing improvement in health as an *objective*, but in this book we delineate between *goal* and *objective* as specialist terms. *Target* is not used here as a specialist term.

Note: National Health Goals refer to non-measureable, non-time-specific goals as described above. National Health *Targets* equate with goals in the sense in which *goal* is used in this book.

Health An important resource for living; physical abilities and social and psychological capacities to achieve one's potential and respond positively to the challenges of the environment. (After Nutbeam.)

Health attitude A view or way of thinking about health or health behaviour. For example, if knowledge refers to the awareness that the rate of breast cancer is high among women who smoke, attitude might refer to the desire to decrease one's chances of contracting cancer as well as the intention to stop smoking.

Health behaviour (health-directed behaviour) Any activity undertaken by an individual with the intention of maintaining, protecting or promoting health, whether or not the activity is effective for that purpose.

For example, an individual may greatly increase their intake of unprocessed bran with the intention of improving their health (e.g. reducing blood cholesterol). Whether or not taking bran affects blood cholesterol levels (and whether or not they take the right sort of bran), this is a health behaviour for that individual.

Note: The reader should understand the distinction between health behaviour (intentional health-directed behaviour) and health-related behaviour, which is not necessarily consciously directed by the individual towards improving health, but which has been identified as affecting health, either positively or negatively.

Using the same example as above, an individual may have been eating bran because they liked it. The fact there is no intention to affect health does not prevent the behaviour from affecting health. In this case valuable calcium is not absorbed, causing osteoporosis. From this perspective, eating too much bran is a health-related behaviour.

Health-related behaviour Any activity undertaken by an individual which has been shown to have a positive or negative effect on health, whether or not such activity is carried out with any intention towards health. (See *health behaviour*.)

Health belief A statement or sense, declared or implied, intellectually and/ or emotionally accepted as true by a person or group. May motivate behaviour related to health (after Green).

Health care costs The most common use of this term is to mean the expenditures associated with a service or programme. These are the historical amounts paid.

Health care costs can also mean the value of the resources used by a service or programme. Some resources may be used but not paid for, e.g. the work of volunteers or the use of the meeting room in the health centre. Health care costs may fall on clients, service providers, the government or health insurance funds. For example, while the stress management group leader works at the health centre and the group meets there, group participants must travel to the centre and pay for the refreshments provided afterwards. Clearly, counting the costs depends on whose viewpoint you take.

Opportunity cost is the value of the resources in their best alternative use. Resources for health care are limited; it is not possible to provide every service or programme that would be beneficial in health terms. So choosing to use resources in one programme rather than another means forgoing the health benefits of the other programme.

From the concept of opportunity cost, it can be seen that the health costs of *not* preventing ill health are the health benefits forgone. These health costs comprise health care costs, that is the resources used in treating ill health (called direct costs), the losses in productivity when people cannot work (called indirect costs) and the value of life and good health (called intangible costs).

Health education Consciously constructed opportunities for learning which are designed to facilitate voluntary changes in behaviour towards a predetermined goal. It is closely associated with disease prevention and involves changing behaviours which have been identified as risk factors for particular diseases. Targets individuals and groups, organizations and communities (after Green).

In the past, *health education* was used to refer to the broad range of initiatives now covered by the term *health promotion*. The term *health education* now tends to refer to educational programmes seeking to bring about voluntary changes in behaviour, but the reader should be aware that the broader meaning is still often used.

Health indicator   Health statistics selected for their capacity to summarize a larger body of statistics or to serve as indirect or proxy measures for a concept that cannot be directly measured (after Murnaghan), e.g. infant mortality rate, life expectancy at birth.

Health indicators purport to measure the health of a population. They are typically expressed as percentages, rates or ratios. Traditionally, health indicators have been seen as a subset of *social indicators*. More recently the distinction has become blurred, as the understanding of health and its concerns has broadened to overlap with social concerns. For example, population age profiles and employment rates are often used as indicators of levels of health. See also *social indicator*.

Health intervention   Any planned action which is aimed at reducing a health problem by intervening in the existing causal chain. An intervention is the sum of all the *strategies*; that is, those events, circumstances or materials which directly involve the target group or the community. An intervention may consist of one strategy, or more than one (see also *programme*).

Health knowledge   The information that an individual has, or has access to, which provides the basis for decisions about health, health behaviour, risk behaviour, and sometimes attitude.

Health problem   Diseases and other conditions or circumstances affecting health which will not be tolerated by an individual or community and which are identified as requiring intervention.

Health professional (health worker)   A person who is employed in the organized health care services. The term health professional covers workers from a wide range of backgrounds but is usually used to describe those who have had formal training in health studies and whose work directly concerns the theory and/or practice of health care or preventive health, as opposed to support personnel. E.g. doctors, nurses, social workers, health educators, physiotherapists, etc.

Health promotion   The process of enabling individuals and communities to increase control over the determinants of health and thereby improve their health (Nutbeam). Health promotion grew out of the *health education* movement, but can now be understood as an umbrella concept which covers health education and a number of other approaches aimed at changing living conditions and lifestyles for the purpose of promoting health.

Health promotion as defined by Green and Anderson consists of a combination of health education plus related organizational, economic and/or environmental supports for behaviour of individuals, groups or communities which is a conducive to health. Under our definition, health promotion need not include education as one of its components. For example, a programme of lobbying the meat and livestock industry to reduce the allowed fat content in meat is a health promotion activity. It may be carried out in conjuction with an education programme but can make a significant impact on health without it.

Health services   Refers to the organized provision of health care by *health professionals*, both in the public and private sectors. Examples: hospitals, community health centres, specialist medical and paramedical services such as podiatry, acupuncture, Red Cross, ENT specialist.

Health status   State of physical and/or mental and/or social functioning. The literature on health status measurement for the most part predates the concern with quality of life, but some measures incorporate aspects now thought of as quality of life.

Health worker—see **health professional**

Incidence   The rate of occurrence of new cases or manifestions of a health problem in a defined population in a given period of time.

Impact evaluation   Follows *evaluability assessment* in the steps of *programme evaluation* and is the first step in testing a completed programme's performance. Impact evaluation is concerned with the immediate effects of the programme, that is its effect on those factors which contribute to or cause the health problem in question. Corresponds to the measurement of programme *objectives*. Should include an assessment of both intended and unintended effects

Intersectoral   In health promotion, health-oriented policy affecting and involving sectors outside health services (such as employment, housing, food production, social care), but usually evolved in collaboration with the health sector. Also used to refer to collaboration between different levels of various sectors—e.g. government health authorities plus local transport authority plus community education.

As an example of an intersectoral programme, consider a heart health programme. This project may involve members of the community in developing community awareness and making community education possible; health professionals in the screening, referral and management of high cholesterol levels in individuals; members of the food retail industries in promoting low-fat foods at point of sale; and agriculture department representatives in producing low-fat meat.

Intervention group (programme group, programme participants, participant group)   Any collection of individuals participating in a health programme or intervention. In most cases the intervention group consists of those who will directly benefit (*target group*) or a subset of this group. In some cases a programme may be directed at one group of people for the benefit of another group. For example, in drug education for parents, the parents are the *intervention group* but the children are the *target group*.

Knowledge—see **health knowledge**

Locus of control   Refers to the extent to which a person believes that their own behaviour influences their health, amongst other important aspects of life, such as career, success, happiness, wealth.

Morbidity   Illness episodes. *Morbidity data* refers to data which describe the prevalence of different diseases and other health problems in the community. The main source of this is hospital admission records which include diagnosis, or reason for admission. Data collected by GPs, health centres, etc. may also be used.

Mortality   Death. *Mortality data* on causes and number of deaths per year are collected by the Registrar General in each State. These are presented as proportions of the population by the Australian Bureau of Statistics.

Need Health needs are understood as being those states, conditions or factors in the community that, if absent, prevent people from achieving optimum physical, mental and social health. This would include such things as minimum provision of basic health services and information, a safe physical environment, good food and housing, productive work and activity and a network of emotionally supportive and stimulating relationships.

When talking about need there is sometimes a conceptual shuffle between defining need as the deficit or problem (for example poor health) and stating the problem in terms of its solution, such as provision of health care. Be conscious of this because what is deemed to be a satisfactory solution to a problem varies between different schools of opinion and across time as technology and views change.

Needs assessment The initial step in planning any health intervention; the process of identifying and analysing the priority health problem and the nature of the *target group*, for the purpose of planning an intervention.

Network A set of relationships which centres on one individual's circle of contacts and branches outward to include relationships between these people, their own unique contacts, and others already in the network.

The professional networks of health workers and the social networks of health consumers are both very important. In health promotion, *social network* refers specifically to the number and types of social relations and links between individuals which may provide access to or mobilization of *social support* for health (after Nutbeam).

Networking In health promotion:
1. building up the quantity and quality of one's relationships;
2. making use of one's social or professional network for the purpose of generating or receiving information or support.

Non-equivalent (of a comparison group) A comparison group whose members cannot be considered as being like the intervention group with respect to member characteristics. This contrasts with the *control group*, where all participants have a chance of being allocated to the control group or the experimental group, and then the groups are termed equivalent groups.

Objective The desired immediate impact of a health promotion programme; an improvement in factors which contribute to the health problem. It is measurable (how much improvement, by when, by whom).

Outcome evaluation The final phase of *programme evaluation* and the second of the two-step process which tests the performance of a programme. Outcome evaluation answers the question of whether a programme has achieved its goal; whether it has been able to reduce the health need or alleviate the problem isolated at the needs assessment stage, and at what cost.

Outcome evaluation corresponds to measurement of programme *goals*, whereas *impact evaluation* corresponds with measurement of programme *objectives*. In this regard outcome evaluation is concerned with longer-term effects than those addressed in impact evaluation.

Perceived health   An individual's interpretation of experiences of health and ill-health within the context of everyday living. This judgement is normally based on available knowledge and information modified by previous experience and social and cultural norms (Nutbeam).

Post-test   Observations or measurements concerning participant's knowledge, attitudes, behaviour, health status etc., taken at or after the conclusion of a health programme. Usually compared with measurements taken before the programme (*Pre-test*) for the purpose of assessing programme effects.

Predisposing factor   Any characteristic of an individual, a community or an environment that predisposes behaviour or other conditions related to health. Includes knowledge, belief and attitude, but may include other factors such as socioeconomic status.

These factors can predispose conditions which lead to ill health, or conditions which lead to good health. For example, lack of knowledge of the sexual transmission of HIV predisposes people to practising unsafe sex.

Prevalence   The proportion of cases or manifestations of a health problem in a defined population at a particular point in time (point prevalence) or occurring during a specified period of time (period prevalence).

Pre-test

1. Observations or measurements concerning participants' knowledge, attitudes, behaviour, health status etc., taken at the start of a health programme. Another test is taken at the completion of the programme (*post-test*) and comparison made in order to evaluate programme effects.

2. Pilot; part of *process evaluation*. Materials to be used in a programme are pre-tested or trialled before being adopted in final form. Leaflets, audio-visuals, questionnaires etc. are presented to a group of people similar to the target group, or to some members of the target group, or other health workers for their reactions and opinions and to test the suitability and acceptability of the material.

Process evaluation   Process evaluation is the first element of programme evaluation. It measures the activity of the programme and who it is reaching. It determines to what extent a programme has been implemented as planned, by measuring (a) *programme reach*, (b) participant satisfaction, (c) implementation of programme activities, (d) performance of materials or other components, (e) ongoing quality assurance.

Process evaluation includes pre-testing of materials or other components of the programme and may lead to the redesign or re-implementation of programme elements. See *formative evaluation*.

Programme   A coherent series of activities, which together make up one strategy or more than one strategy, carried out with a group of participants for the purpose of improving the health status of the target group. This can be individual behaviour change, or environmental, legislative or other change. A programme is usually planned in response to an established health *need*.
   Note: 1. Sometimes programme is used synonomously with *intervention*.
             2. The literature also uses intervention programme (e.g. Nutbeam) for what is referred to here as programme.

Programme evaluation   Assessment of programme effectiveness; the process of determining the value or degree of success of a programme in achieving predetermined goals and objectives. Also involves the assessment of unintended effects.

Programme group   Those people to whom a programme is delivered; the participants of the programme. Equates with *experimental group* in a research setting. (See *intervention group*.)

Programme planning   This is the second step in the planning and evaluation cycle, following *needs assessment*. The process of articulating what you are trying to achieve with your programme, why you are doing it and how you will go about it. Includes setting *goals* and *objectives*, selecting *strategies* and designing *activities* for the programme.

Programme reach   A measure of the extent to which a campaign or programme has made contact with the target group. This involves one of two comparisons:
   (a)   how many people were involved in a programme, compared with the number of people known or estimated to belong to the *target group*;
   (b)   how many people who, when surveyed, can recall and/or describe a given campaign message, compared with the total number of people surveyed.

Quality of life Some writers use this term to refer to subjective assessment of function and satisfaction independent of health status. Others, particularly in the medical/clinical literature, use it to cover health-related quality of life, meaning aspects of the outcome or side-effects of disease or its treatment other than the signs of the disease itself.

Qualitative data   Data which describe the range of response and variation between responses but do not record frequency of response. Cannot be used with tests of statistical significance.

Quantitative data   Data which are recorded as frequency of response; response options may be categorical (e.g. male/female); ordinal (e.g. never/sometimes/often) or numerical (number of cigarettes smoked per day). Hypotheses may be supported or rejected by applying tests of statistical significance to quantitative data.

Quasli-experimental   Any research design looking for effects which is not a true experiment. That is, in quasi-experimental designs, participants are not randomly allocated to the experimental or programme group.

Some quasi-experimental designs are:
a)   non-equivalent groups; pre-test and post-test
b)   single group; time series,
c)   non-equivalent groups; time series.

Randomized controlled trial (equivalent groups design)   Random assignment gives all participants an equal chance of being allocated to the *experimental group* or the *control group*. The groups are compared by *pre-testing* and *posttesting*, or by *time series* testing.

This design is the 'true experiment'. It is considered the strongest design for demonstrating causality.

Reinforcing factor   Any reward or punishment or any feedback following or anticipated as a consequence of health behaviour (after Green).

Reliability   A property of questionnaires, surveys or any other measurement tool. Expresses the degree to which the same score is produced on repeated measures with a given instrument, in the absence of any real change. Repeated measures refers to measurements taken with the same instrument either by the same person at different times (test-retest reliability) or by different people (inter-observer reliability).

Resources
1. In terms of programme planning—commitments of finances, staff time, expertise and energy and emotional commitments required to run a health programme. Usually considered from the point of view of the providers of the programme but may include resources from within the community or the programme participants.
2. In terms of the health care consumer—personal, educational, financial, social and political capabilities to improve one's own situation, or to obtain help in doing so.

Response rate   The number of people who complete and return a survey compared with the number of people who were sent survey forms.

Risk factor   Any aspect of behaviour, society or the environment which is directly linked to a health problem in an established or proposed causal pathway. A health problem may have one or more than one risk factor; e.g. smoking and elevated levels of serum cholsterol are both risk factors for heart disease. (See *risk marker*.)

Risk marker (risk indicator)   Any characteristic which signals where a problem is occurring and identifies individuals or groups as being at risk of a particular health problem. Risk markers are associated with the occurrence of the problem, but are not necessarily thought to cause the problem. Examples include age and sex. Risk markers usually cannot be changed or are not appropriate targets for intervention, but should be considered in planning the sort of intervention most likely to succeed.

For example, having English as one's mother tongue identifies those at higher risk of heart disease, but the language spoken is not thought to cause disease.

The reader should be aware that some authors do not discriminate between causally related and associative factors, using contributing factor or risk factor for both. But this can lead to problems in identifying which factors need intervention.

Sample   A selected subset of a population; may be random or non-random and may be representative or non-representative (Last).

Self-efficacy   Refers to the expectation that a person has concerning whether a given behaviour can be successfully performed by them (e.g. quitting smoking, managing asthma). Theory first put forward by Albert Bandura.

Site (setting)   The physical or institutional environment in which a strategy component and its activities are employed, e.g. school, hospital, community.

For example, the education of children concerning pedestrian crossings may take place at the school and in the home.

Social epidemiology The study of the distribution and determinants of ill-health, with particular and sophisticated reference to social phenomena and dependence on sociological theory. Social epidemiology emphasizes that some health problems, such as depression, may have social causes, and may respond to a social solution (after Nutbeam).

Social indicator A directly measurable variable used as a measure of the wellbeing of individuals in a community, which is not directly measurable. For example, population age distribution, income levels, educational attainment, house or car ownership, life expectancy.

Traditionally, health indicators have been seen as a subset of social indicators. (See *health indicator*).

Social marketing Social marketing sees the consumers of health services as clients of interventions, and applies marketing principles to the promotion of products beneficial to health (which may be ideas, causes, behaviours or services). These principles can be summarized as producing the right product at the right price at the right place with right promotion, in response to the market's (or the target group's) needs and wants (after Lefebre and Flora).

Social support Social support is known to have a direct and positive effect upon health and wellbeing and is also known to act as a buffer against stressful life events. There are different types of assistance which an individual is able to obtain from people with whom they come into contact. Four types of social support are usually identified. These are emotional support, instrumental support (which includes the provision of money, goods and services, and assistance with everyday tasks), informational support, and appraisal (meaning feedback to the individual about their identity, personality and behaviour).

Social support is assessed according to whether it is potentially available (perceived support) or whether it was actually received. Its quality and adequacy can also be evaluated.

Strategy In health promotion, the type of approach used to effect desired changes in *predisposing, enabling* or *reinforcing factors*, as set down in the *sub-objectives*. A sub-objective may have more than one strategy. The main strategies are education, organization, legislation and regulation.

Strategy components The practical applications of a chosen strategy to the intervention situation concerned. For example, given the objective of improving children's diet, a strategy of education might generate strategy components including: posters of healthy foods displayed at school; information sent home to parents on preparing nutritious meals.

These activities might be supported by a strategy of regulation, which might include strategy components such as regulating the school canteen menu to include nutritious foods.

Sub-objective Any desired change in a *predisposing, enabling* or *reinforcing* *factor*. It is measurable. Sub-objectives represent the component parts of the objective.

Survey An investigation in which information is systematically collected from a population sample, e.g. face-to-face inquiry, self-completed questionnaire or telephone survey.

Target group Those members of a community for whose benefit a health goal is constructed and a health intervention carried out. These people are usually the programme participants or *intervention group* although in some cases the participants might be another group of people who will pass on the benefit to the target group. For example, a parent drug education programme may be aimed at reducing drug abuse in children, in which case the children are the target group and the parents are the intervention group.

Time series design Modification of the *pre-test-post-test* design. A series of measurements is made on an experimental group (and sometimes on the control group) on several occasions before and after the programme is run. This design aims to compare the impact of the programme with any unsolicited changes or existing trends in the participating group.

Total environment In health promotion, all identifiable aspects of the social, economic and physical environment which may influence the health of individuals or groups (after Nutbeam).

Users (evaluation users) Those people or bodies that will make use of programme evaluations for the purposes of health planning and resource allocation. (See also *decision makers*.)

Validity A property of questionnaires, surveys, or any other research measurement tool. Expresses the degree to which the tool measures what it purports to measure; for example, to what extent a questionnaire can be a valid measure of smoking status.

References

Bandura A. Self-efficacy: towards a unifying theory of behavioral change. *Psychological Review* 1977;84:191–215.

Green LW, Anderson CL. *Community Health*. St Louis: Times Mirror/Mosby 1986; especially, pp 512–520.

Green LW, Lewis FM. *Measurement and Evaluation In Health Education and Health Promotion*. Palo Alto: Mayfield Publishing, 1986; especially pp 360–367.

Last JM. *A Dictionary of Epidemiology* Oxford: Oxford University Press, 1983.

Lefebvre RC, Flora JA. Social marketing and public health intervention. *Health Education Quarterly* 1988;15:299–315.

Murnaghan JH. Health Indicators and Information systems for the year 2000. *Annual Review of Public Health* 1981;2:299–361.

Nutbeam D. Health promotion glossary. *Health Promotion* 1986;1:113–127.

Annotated Bibliography

JOURNAL ARTICLES

Needs Assessment

The concept of social need
Jonathan Bradshaw. *New Society* 1972;19:640–643.

The concept of need is complex, and can be divided into four dimensions. The advisability of basing decisions on each is discussed.

1. The *normative* need of a community is defined here not as the norm, but as a level of service which is deemed to be a desirable standard for the whole community. It is worth as much as its deemer. Establishing a normative need is more a statement of policy than a needs assessment measurement.

2. The *felt* (attitudinal) need is that expressed by a community. This is a good measure, but subject to many biases. Sometimes, people don't know what they want: they only want what they know.

3. The *expressed* (behavioural) need is measured by counting the number of people using or demanding a service. The limitations of this measure are obvious: people may not know about a service; they may be isolated from it; they may see putting their names on waiting lists as a waste of time. The reasons for which people do *not* use a service are often important indicators of need.

4. The *comparative* need is the extent to which a community has a lower provision of services than a comparable community. Like normative need, this notion may be helpful to policy makers but is of less use to researchers.

The second half of the paper consists of a discussion of the implications of the various combinations of needs which a community may experience. In this discussion, rows of four symbols are used. The fourth is labelled 'comparative need', but actually represents *supply* which is, in a sense, the opposite of comparative need.

This is a seminal paper. Its terminology has now, deservedly, become widespread.

Issues in the measurement of 'community need'
Elery Hamilton-Smith. *Australian Journal of Social Issues* 1975; 10(1): 35–45.

This paper more or less includes Bradshaw's, along with plenty of examples and a more comprehensive discussion of how to base planning decisions on a needs assessment. A standard of normative need is always nice but rarely available, and must usually be synthesized from felt, expressed and comparative needs data.

Since the process of investigating a community's felt needs exposes it to new knowledge and new aspirations, it's important for a researcher to try to involve the community in programmes of change or, at least, provide feedback about how the research is using the community's input.

The relationship of needs assessment to policy setting is very well expressed in this article.

Assessing the need for a needs assessment

Ron Wutchiett, Davin Egan, Susan Kohaut, Howard J. Markman and Kenneth I. Pargament. *Journal of Community Psychology* 1984;12:53–60.

An evaluation of a programme's impact can be preceded by an evaluability assessment, to make sure that the time-consuming impact evaluation will produce some usable results (positive or negative). In the same way, it's a good idea to check before embarking on a needs assessment that the results will be used for something.

If a needs assessment is only going to waste resources and create an impression of activity but not enhance services, then it should be cancelled or postponed.

The things to look for in agency administrators and service planners include:
1. their attitudes towards needs data which they already have;
2. their attitudes towards future needs assessments;
3. the types of information which they want;
4. their willingness to use the results ⎫ investigated using
5. their ability to use the results ⎭ hypothetical results.

In the example recounted here, the authors found that agency administrators viewed assessment data primarily as a means to justify existing services. Rather than conduct a new needs assessment, the authors asked each agency to reanalyse the existing data, and encouraged an interest in community needs as a whole as opposed to those within each agency's current realm of operations.

Mental health needs assessment: beware of false promises

David Royse and Kenneth Drude. *Community Mental Health Journal* 1982; 18(2): 97–106

A practical paper by authors who are concerned about the difficulty of basing planning decisions on needs assessments. Unfortunately, there is no gold standard to which needs assessments can aspire. Needs assessment techniques are so variable (not only in quality but also in aims and focus) that most researchers have resorted to combining several techniques in the hope that the various assessments will build up a picture of true need. This is helpful, but makes policy decisions even more difficult as there is no systematic procedure for relating the data from one approach to the data from the next.

The situation would be improved by standardization—if assessments all used the same instruments, they would at least be comparable to each other.

The authors foresee expert committees to choose the best standard assessment tools. In the meantime, they make some recommendations of their own for mental health professionals

Goals and priorities in prevention: the challenge of chronic disease and disability

G. Goldstein. *Community Health Studies* 1983;7(1):54–59.

An interesting paper on the philosophy of health planning.

The author argues against the World Health Organisation's definition of health as

> *a positive state of mental, physical and social well-being and not merely the absence of disease or infirmity.*

The question at issue is not just whether the definition should be phrased positively or negatively, but also exactly what qualities a person should have in order to be considered healthy.

On the slightly different question of how to set goals and priorities in health planning, the author prefers the negative definition of health as the absence of disease because reductions in disease are easily quantifiable.

The consequences of such an approach include an expansion of effective preventive interventions, the formulation of a minimum standard of personal health care and explicit rather than implicit rationing of health services. If our health concerns are chosen according to criteria like invalidism and inability to work (alongside the traditional concern for mortality), coronary heart disease and cancer are rivalled by chronic problems like neurosis and arthritis.

The inadequacy of needs assessments of the elderly

Leslie S. Larau and Leonard F. Heumann. *The Gerontologist* 1982;22(3): 324–330.

An appraisal of the needs assessments carried out by agencies which provide services to senior citizens in the US.

Although the importance of needs assessment was widely recognized, only 10% of the agencies surveyed were able to present reports of needs assessments, and three-quarters of these were considered inadequately conducted.

Most of the recommendations in this article are specific to the problems of the elderly and the resources available in the US, but the way in which the assessments were evaluated is exemplary. The authors examined:

1.   the sources of data (random survey, key informants, group process, secondary data, secondary findings, service user records and service request records);

2. the use of descriptive variables (age, household size, etc.);
3. the use of needs indicators (current use, expressed desire and inferrences drawn from data about lack of services);
4. the comprehensiveness of each study;
5. the matching of needs to existing services.

A community's health education needs must be defined

Malcolm S. Weinstein and Dewey Evans. *Health Education* 1983; Fall: 2–7.

A high-level look at how to assess the needs of a community. The authors give us a number of methods for eliciting information about community needs from both health service consumers and health service providers. These are: random consumer surveys, key informant surveys, health fairs, small nominal group workshops, meetings of consumer groups, the Delphi technique of repeatedly refined questionnaires, government vital statistics, clinical records, institutional records, specific disease registers, records of notification, records of reiterated episodes of illness, resource profiles from agencies and inter-agency meetings.

A rough timetable is given for using all this information. The assessment process may be cyclic as community needs are constantly changing.

The authors argue that health educators have two roles in needs assessment. The first is researcher (to collect information). The second is community developer (to help communities to identify, and work towards, solutions to problems).

Alternate methods for health priority assessment

F. Douglas Scutchfield. *Journal of Community Health* 1975;1(1):29–38.

This paper illustrates four methods of needs assessment: nominal group technique, community diagnosis, random community survey and priority ratings by health professionals. All four methods gave very similar results when applied to a rural community in the US.

The rationale of each method is explained, although not enough detail is given to let the reader reproduce the techniques or even interpret the results.

The author suggests that there is a discrepancy between the experts' interests in specific health problems (e.g., car accidents) and consumers' emphasis on resource problems (e.g., a lack of community medical services).

Processes of Consultation and Planning

Participation in community intervention design

Donald D. Davis. *American Journal of Community Psychology* 1982;10(4): 429–445.

Argues that community participation is necessary to ensure that programmes reflect the diversity of values within a community, and to promote community control of interventions. Five participation methods are described: public hearings, surveys, Delphi technique, dialectical scanning and nominal group technique.

The author suggests that different sorts of participation strategies be used according to different stages of intervention planning. For example, surveys and Delphi technique are recommended for needs assessment and nominal group technique is recommended for selecting strategies or methods of intervention and for evaluation.

This is an excellent appraisal of the purpose and methods of participation. The article is written from the perspective of the community psychologist, but this should not put off readers from other disciplines.

Need and demand in the making of planning decisions in the evaluation of health and welfare services

A. Stevenson and W. Chew. In Senate Select Committee on Social Welfare. *Through A Glass Darkly: Evaluation in Australian Health and Welfare Services*, vol. 2. Canberra: AGPS, 1979.

A sociological and political critique of needs assessment and evaluation in Australian health and welfare services. Since such services are altruistic, they are measured against the yardstick of aiming to help people fairly (that is, regardless of the people's ability to champion their own needs).

Consumer participation in services is praised. Services are usually planned to fit in with lobbying interests, including the opinions of experts. Relatively inarticulate consumers are given relatively little power. A solution to this problem is for planners to carry out careful, qualitative assessments of felt need, and to allow consumer evaluations to shape the development of their programmes. (If a service isn't related to a felt need, people won't be motivated to use it.)

This long paper makes many other interesting points about social planning.

The nominal group technique: a health education strategy

Larry Laufman, Nicholas K. Iammarino and Armin D. Weinberg. *Health Education*, 1981; January/February: 17–19.

A short article on how to use nominal group technique in a short meeting.

The virtue of nominal group technique is that it allows a group to clarify its decisions without being dominated by excessively loud individuals. Each member of the group lists his/her ideas (in this case, concerns about health); the lists are pooled, and each member ranks his/her priorities.These ranks are then analysed.

This digestible account gives precise guidelines for applying the technique under the time constraints of a school classroom.

A group process model for problem identification and program planning

André L. Delbecq and Andrew H. Van de Ven. *Journal of Applied Behavioural Science* 1971;7(4):466–492.

This article recommends a long, organized procedure which pre-empts later conflicts of interest by involving consumers, experts, administrators and resource controllers before and during the programme planning phase. The procedure, which includes nominal group technique, is described in great detail (right down to the sizes of cards written on in meticulously timed meetings).

This article is useful in that it gives a precise description of the process which the authors advocate, but it is doubtful that many people would want to replicate it exactly.

The Utilization of Evaluation Findings

Enhancing the utilization of evaluation findings
William R. Tash and Gerald J. Stahler. *Community Mental Health Journal* 1982;18:180–189.

A constructive examination of the problem of under-utilization of evaluation findings, with good recommendations and broad implications (not just for mental health). An exemplary evaluation is presented as an illustration of the theory, which involves five suggestions for the recommendations which come out of an evaluation.

1. Identify specific user audiences and tailor recommendations to these groups.

2. Formulate recommendations collaboratively with the user audiences.

3. Direct specific recommendations towards the development of a broader policy and programme model.

4. Assess the impact of the recommendations over time.

5. Make an effort to present recommendations in an empathic way.

This article is well written and profitable to all evaluators who liaise with decision makers.

Evaluation research in the political context
Carol H. Weiss. In Streunig EL and Guttentag M (eds).
Handbook of Evaluation Research, Vol 1. Beverly Hills: Sage Publications, 1975.

A well-written and sensible look at the effects of politics on evaluation.

Most of the political problems of evaluators are due to the fact that neither politicians nor administrators will necessarily agree with evaluators about what is rational. Evaluators may have to make a big effort to address the values of the decision makers who will use the evaluation reports.

Policy makers are concerned with political compromises involving interest groups (including, but not solely, their consciences and the voting or vocal public). What evaluation research can do is clarify what the compromises involve in terms of health promotion outcomes.

For example, because statements of goals are designed to secure support, they set extravagent levels of expectation. A good evaluation will show which goals were evaluable (the evaluable programme model), which were actually worked towards (process evaluation) and which were achieved (impact and outcome evaluation).

Implementing a pluralistic approach to evaluation in health education
Robin Means and Randall Smith. *Policy and Politics* 1988;16(1):17–28.

A detailed case study of an alcohol education programme and its evaluation. The authors explain and illustrate the fact that it is not always possible to make an evaluation conform to an experimental or quasi-experimental design. To make matters worse, the policy makers' goals are usually not unambiguously clear before the programme is started (if ever), making evaluability assessment difficult.

One solution to this problem, resources permitting, is for the evaluators to take a *pluralistic* approach. This means that they document and evaluate several different concepts of success simultaneously. Pluralistic evaluation faces political complications, especially in process evaluation and particularly in high-profile programmes. On the other hand, it can be an excellent solution to inter- agency conflict.

Being mostly an account of the political struggles of one project, this article is useful for those whose programmes' goals are unclear or dubiously imposed from outside.

How evaluation findings can be integrated into program decision making
Judith Blanton and Sam Alley. *Community Mental Health Journal* 1978; 14(3):239–247.

A broadly applicable paper (not specific to mental health) which deals with ways of integrating the findings of evaluation studies into the process of decision making, particularly for evaluations which are conducted within an organization which will then have scope for improving its operations.

This article presents valuable suggestions on eliciting data and presenting evaluation results. For example, recommendations must be translated into behavioural or structural changes in order to influence programme efficiency and effectiveness. Programme staff (including decision makers) must hear and understand the information, be willing to accept its validity and be able and willing to make the recommended changes.

Many useful strategies for overcoming cognitive resistance (due to lack of understanding) and affective resistance (due to lack of motivation) are discussed.

A user-focused model for the utilization of evaluation
Terry Connolly and Alan L. Porter. *Evaluation and Program Planning* 1980;3:131–140.

The present under-utilization of evaluation findings is partly traceable to their failure to directly address the information needs of an individual decision maker. This article is concerned with knowledge for the sake of action rather than for the sake of understanding. Although evaluations which are disseminated in the usual academic way will have some impact on decision makers, the authors hypothesize that utilization will be higher for 'user-focused' evaluations—those produced in response to a specific informational need of a specific decision maker.

Many implications of this user-focused model are explained—for example, the importance of formative evaluation, including both process evaluation and evaluability assessment. Some of the recommendations would damage the scientific validity of the evaluation; fortunately, the user-focused model is not presented as the only model, but merely in order to 'extend the repertoire of evaluation options'.

Whether evaluation—whether utilization

O. Lynn Deniston. *Evaluation and Program Planning* 1980;3:91–94.

Evaluation is defined here as 'measurement, coupled with comparison of the obtained count or score to a criterion or standard'. For example, a good research question is, 'How wide is your chair?' . . . the equivalent evaluation question is, 'Is your chair wide enough to sit on?'

Evaluation is called for whenever a new programme is constructed. The results of such evaluations are always utilized to some extent, but sometimes only by the evaluator and not by the decision makers.

Having thus clarified the issue of under-utilization, the author makes some brief remarks about the desirability of evaluation being conducted by all those involved in research and programme planning and implementation, rather than by isolated, professional evaluators.

Study Design

Different approaches to the evaluation of programs and services

Robyn Robinson. *Australian Psychologist* 1984;19(2):147–161.

An overview of the development of the discipline of health promotion evaluation. Some of the disagreements between evaluation experts are neatly explained by their historical and political contexts and their differences in terminology.

In addition to a well-written history, we have the author's thoughts on the purposes of evaluation and three major types of evaluation design: the experimental model (including quasi-experimental designs), the goal attainment model, and the qualitative 'elucidation' models (non-experimental methods reminiscent of the anthropological approach).

This article is highly recommended to anyone interested in the competing concepts of evaluation.

The feasibility and desirability of experimental methods in evaluation

Nick L. Smith. *Evaluation and Program Planning* 1980;3:251–256.

A marvellously pertinent and sensible article which examines the contention that it is essential for evaluation designs to fit the mould of the scientific, randomized, experimental study. This is considered under two headings: 'Are experimental designs feasible in evaluation?' and 'Are experimental designs desirable in evaluation?'

Pros and cons to these questions are carefully tabulated. The author suggests that experimental designs are usually feasible, but that we should shun a dogmatic answer to the question of their desirability, and answer instead, 'It depends'. Fortunately, we are given thoughtful advice on what factors it depends on, and advised, if in doubt, to adopt a causal, experimental approach, at least as part of the evaluation.

How to evaluate health promotion

Lawrence W. Green. *Hospitals* 1979; October: 106–108.

A short article which attempts to establish a hierarchy of evaluation designs.
1. The historical, record-keeping approach.
2. The 'stop everything' inventory approach.
3. The comparative approach.
4. The controlled comparison (the quasi-experimental design).
5. The controlled experimental approach.
6. The full-blown, double-blind, randomized, controlled trial.

Very little advice is offered on how to choose between these designs. For more help, see the previous article.

Qualitative methods for evaluative research in health education programs

Partricia Dolan Mullen and Donald Iverson. *Health Education* 1982; May/June: 11–18.

Health promotion programmes always have both quantitative and qualitative aspects, and so should their evaluations. Even measurement tools, which are quantitative by nature, should not be used without a good qualitative understanding of the construct which they measure.

Qualitative, unfocused enquiries can supplement quantitative evaluation designs in several ways:

1. by picking up effects outside the scope of the predetermined programme objectives;

2. by suggesting which parts of the programme might be generalizable to which other populations;

3. by subjectively improving the match between the experimental and control groups in non-randomized studies;

4. by explaining results through analyses of the processes at work.

Wise advice is given on when to make the main study method qualitative, although no examples or reasons are given to convince us that we should ever completely ignore quantitative methods.

Towards more rigorous evaluation of health promotion programmes
Neville Owen and Christina Lee. *Australian Psychologist* 1986;21:79–91.

The authors suggest a chain of research and evaluation activities which has the potential to improve the quality of public policy. The recommended steps are:
1. basic laboratory research;
2. controlled intervention trial;
3. trials in field settings under normal (other than ideal) conditions;
4. self-help, mass media and minimal intervention programmes;
5. changes in public policy.

There is often a gap in the chain where step 3 should be.

Face-to-face methods of behaviour change need to be adapted to suit the mass media. Some of the concerns about very-large-scale health promotion programmes are discussed here—in particular, the importance of long-term follow-up of participants, bearing in mind that a transient change in behaviour would rarely improve a population's health.

The commercial advertising style of much mass media promotion is denigrated as it emphasizes awareness over behaviour and the short-term impact over the long-term.

Evaluability Assessment

Evaluability assessment: avoiding types III and IV errors
John W. Scanlon, Pamela Harris, Joe N. Nay, Richard E. Schmidt and John D. Waller. In G. R. Gilbert and P. J. Conklin (eds). *Evaluation Management: A Source Book of Readings*. Charlottesville: U.S. Civil Service Commission, 1971.

An interesting article which extends the old ideas of type I error (identifying an effect which doesn't really exist) and type II error (failing to discover something which does really exist). Two new kinds of error are defined: type III error, measuring something which does not exist; and type IV error, measuring something which is of no importance.

Evaluability assessment is portrayed as the way to avoid these errors, and its rationale is explained, as is the difference between the rhetorical programme model and the evaluable programme model.

Examples cover every type of evaluable project *except* health promotion, but the authors' ideas are very general and easy to apply to a health promotion programme.

Evaluating programs on drug and alcohol related problems
Arie Rotem and Susan Irvine. *Australian Alcohol/Drug Review* 1985; 4:181–186.

A quick overview, with checklists, of the whole evaluation process. Don't be thrown off by the title: the entire article is applicable to all types of programme. The terminology used is different from ours, but easily translatable.

Rotem and Irvine recommend a careful balance between evaluation by field-workers and external evaluation. They also plead that evaluators should bear in mind which problems are *important* as well as which are easy to solve.

Pretesting: a positive approach to evaluation
Andie L. Knutson. *Public Health Reports* 1952;67:699–703.

This article recommends two steps to be carried out in the early stages of a health education programme.

1. A review of the planning process, including:
   a) the identification of the needs of the community;
   b) an explicit agreement on the objectives of the programme;
   c) a choice of methods;
   d) a check that the information to be passed on is accurate.
2. A 'pretest'. This determines whether the programme is likely to achieve its objectives. A short checklist of conditions for a successful programme is given.

Although somewhat vague, the article serves as a reminder of several points which could be considered before the design of an intervention is finalized.

Aspects of Measurement

Choosing measures of health status for individuals in general populations.
John E. Ware, Jr., Robert H. Brook, Allyson R. Davies and Kathleen N. Lohr. *American Journal of Public Health* 1981;71(6):620–625.

A guide to how to choose a measure of health.

The authors suggest that the health of an ill population (e.g., people admitted to a hospital ward) should be measured in terms of disease, whereas most populations are quite healthy and are better covered by measures of physical and mental wellbeing. Social factors should be measured separately: they often *cause* ill health but they don't *constitute* ill health.

A health measure should be: practical to use; easy to understand and interpret; reliable; valid; not too much of a burden on the respondent; and (usually) cheap.

Provided it meets all these criteria, a good measure need not be objective. Sadly, no examples of good measures are given.

Community competence: a positive approach to needs assessment
Jean Goeppinger and A. J. Baglioni, Jr. *American Journal of Community Psychology* 1985;13:507–523.

Argues that needs assessment should focus on a community's strengths as well as its needs. This article represents the first attempt to come up with a measure of community competence or strength of identity and capacity to deal with its own problems.

A community of competent individuals is not necessarily a competent community; it must have features of its own. Eight dimensions of community competence are proposed:
1. commitment;
2. community participation;
3. clarity of situational definitions;
4. articulateness;
5. effective communication;
6. conflict management;
7. management of relations with the world at large;
8. machinery for facilitating participant interaction and decision making.

Four hundred and thirty-three rural Americans were surveyed by telephone to determine whether these dimensions really did represent independent factors. A copy of the instrument is included in the article.

Social support measurement

Charles H. Tardy. *American Journal of Community Psychology* 1985;13(2): 187–202.

Social support is becoming increasingly recognized as a factor involved (directly or indirectly) in determining health status. This is a very useful review of seven measures that have been developed. Each reflects a different interpretation of the vital ingredients of social support.

Each measure is reviewed in terms of:
1. whether it measures the subject's *use* of the support which is available;
2. whether it is only the support network which is described or whether the subject's *satisfaction* with it is also assessed;
3. the *type* of support which is available (e.g., emotional, financial).

Two promising measures of health education program outcomes and asthmatic children

Kathy F. Green and Case Kolff. *Journal of School Health* 1980; August:332–336.

An article dealing with ways of measuring subjects' attitudes about health. Two scales are discussed: the health locus of control scale and the Piers-Harris Children's Self-Concept Scale. Both are found to be reliable instruments for measuring effective educational goals.

Preventive intervention during the perinatal and infancy periods: overview and guidelines for evaluation

Bernard J. Shuman and Frank Masterpasqua. *Prevention in Human Services* 1981;1(1/2):41–57.

A highly specialized article, useful for those involved in perinatal interventions intended to improve early development.

Four measurable dimensions of *social competence* are:
1. physical health;

2. cognitive development, e.g. developmental quotient (DQ);

3. social/emotional development, e.g. Ainsworth's scale of infant attachment;

4. achievement, e.g. Caldwell's Cooperative Preschool Inventory.

IQ may by used to measure *intellectual development*.

This article abounds in references to useful psychological measurement tools.

Goal Attainment Scaling

An exploration of health counseling and goal attainment scaling in health education programs

John A. Bonaguro, Mauren McLaughlin and Karen Sussman. *Journal of School Health* 1984;54:403–406

For a health promoter, the beauty of goal attainment scaling is that it is tailored to each subject in such a way that its very use is liable to have a positive impact on behaviour (although this means that the results will only be generalizable if goal attainment scaling itself is considered part of the intervention).

This article presents a good example of the use of goal attainment scaling during process evaluation, followed by impact evaluation using both goal attainment scaling and an independent test (the Hare Self-Esteem Scale).

An evaluator who uses goal attainment scaling gives a short list of behaviours to be monitored. Behaviour priorities and attainment goals are individually assigned to each subject. This means that the goal attainment scores of two subjects are not comparable to each other; but the scores of a group after an intervention can be compared to the scores of the same group before the intervention, giving a good impact measure.

The study evaluated here seems to show the attractiveness of health counselling as a supplement to ordinary school health education.

Goal attainment scaling: a critical review

Solomon Cytrynbaum, Yigal Ginath, Joel Birdwell and Lauren Brandt. *Evaluation Quarterly* 1979;3(1):5–40.

This intelligent article includes a good summary of what goal attainment scaling is in its several forms. It makes explicit the distinct choices:

1. to use goal attainment scaling for impact evaluation; or

2. to use goal attainment scaling as part of an intervention (changing people's behaviour).

The value of using goal attainment scaling as an impact measure depends on its reliability and validity. The authors have an admirable grasp of the methodological theory involved, but they can find no conclusive evidence on these questions.

In a large pool of studies purporting to use goal attainment scaling, there is a horrendous incidence of deviance from the original goal attainment scaling model. Some of this (such as joint goal setting) is a useful broadening of the technique; some, however, consists of ad hoc changes leading to invalid evaluation.

Case Studies in Evaluation

An evaluation of a community outreach program

Donald E. Miskiman. *American Journal of Community Psychology* 1979; 7:71–77.

A gripping article which shows how process evaluation can be conducted even in a setting which makes an evaluator armed with a questionnaire scared of bodily violence.

Project Help is an outreach preventive programme developed by a group of religious and social workers in Edmonton, Canada. It provides a contact point for young people, and a bridge between its clients and essential services (spiritual, emotional, medical, legal). The clients, who are generally engaged in a variety of criminal activities, are recruited simply by word of mouth. Project Help is run in bars and coffee houses.

Since undercover law enforcement agents are also found in these places, the clients are inclined to mistrust strangers. Process evaluation was necessarily conducted in a structured but very informal way, with interviewers gratuitously striking up conversations with bar patrons and then rushing to the lavatories to write up their interviewees' replies. These replies were combined with the observations of Project Help staff.

This article reaches the heartening conclusion that the unorthodox process evaluation was able to reveal high levels of consumer awareness of the project and its objectives.

A randomized controlled trial of an information booklet for hypertensive patients in general practice.

C. J. Watkins, A. O. Papacosta, S. Chinn and J. Martin. *Journal of the RCGP* 1987;37:548–550.

An example of a highly quantitative approach to evaluation which produces very precise results with good internal validity at the expense of breadth of vision.

The information booklet referred to in the title was designed to improve patient participation in the management of hypertension. One year after receiving the booklets, only 23% of the patients were still using them. No process evaluation was done to ensure that the booklets were being read or to find out what the patients thought of them.

The impact was marginal: knowledge about hypertension was only slightly higher in those who had received the booklet than in those who had not. The outcome was negative: those who had read the booklet had approximately the same average blood pressure as the controls.

Cigarette smoking and drug use in schoolchildren:
III—evaluation of a smoking prevention education
programme
D. M. Lloyd, H. M. Alexander, R. Callcott, A. J. Dobson, D. L.
O'Connell and S. R. Leeder. *International Journal of Epidemiology* 1983;
12:51–58.

An outcome evaluation of a badly-run programme which failed to achieve its
goals (to reduce the number of 10-to-12-year-olds who took up smoking over
the period of a year).

The evaluation design was a randomized, controlled trial. Confidential, self-
administered questionnaires were completed by children before a $13^1\!/\!2$ hour
educational programme, and again a year later. Parents and teachers were also
surveyed for information about the children's demographic and social contexts.

The teachers' questionnaires also gave process evaluation information, but
only *after* the intervention. Those teachers who had not implemented the
programme fully obtained the worst results; only those who had implemented
it well did better than the control teachers who did not use it at all.

The authors conclude that health education must have better support, if it
is to be effective. They found that behaviour changes were generally unrelated
to knowledge changes, but closely related to changes in attitude.

Evaluating the impact of prevention programmes aimed at children
Elane M. Nuehring, Harvey A. Abrams, David F. Fike and Ellen
Fritsche Ostrowsky. *Social Work Research and Abstract* 1983:19:11–18.

Two examples of impact evaluation are given, along with some theorizing
about primary prevention in mental health. The distinction between impact
evaluation and outcome evaluation is well presented here.

The first example study was conducted by an agency which, with a small
amount of outside consultation, developed and validated its own impact
measures and achieved not only an analysis of the success of the programme
but also improvements to the programme and increased involvement and
morale for the staff.

The second study illustrates the use of the goal attainment scaling system of
evaluation, with similar results.

The details in this article are for those interested in social work or mental
health, but the outlines of exemplary impact evaluation on a small budget
might cheer up any reader.

Other Issues in Evaluation
Potential uses and misuses of education in health promotion and disease prevention
John P. Allegrante. *Teachers College Record* 1988, 86(2):359–373.

A marvellous overview of the history and concepts underlying the movement
towards health promotion.

Four factors influence health: biology, the environment, lifestyle and medical care. The historical foundation of health promotion lies in the enormous cost of curative medicine and, for rich countries, its inability to deal with the environmental and lifestyle factors which cause so much of their mortality.

Health promotion can address these problems, but it will need to include more than just exhortations to individuals to change their behaviour. Some of the responsibility for preventing disease can be taken by individuals on their own behalves, but a more powerful preventive approach is to consider the 'upstream' manufacturers of illness: the cultural, social, economic and political elements which obstruct health promotion.

Although not on the compulsory homework list as it is not strictly about evaluation, this is an excellent, first-principles summary of philosophical Competency-based program evaluation: a contingency approach

Competency-based program evaluation: a contingency approach
Marcus D. Ingle and Rudi Klauss. *Evaluation and Program Planning* 1981; 3:277–287.

What types of professional competency should an evaluator have?

The authors believe that a team approach to evaluation is best, with different skills being called for from different members of the team and for different programmes. Four broad categories of competency are identified: technical (including study design and analysis), personal/interpersonal (including communication and ethics), administrative and policy analysis. This analysis highlights the need for the evaluator to have skills other than research methodology.

Methodologic problems in the evaluation of self-management programs
W. James Popham and Elanna S. Yalow. *Journal of Allergy and Clinical Immunolology* 1983;73(5):581–590.

A variety of evaluation topics is considered in the light of the power of evaluation to *improve programmes* as well as *prove* their results In the authors' experience, an emphasis on improvement is the most potent way of reaching health goals.

Suggestions are made on the nature of evaluation, the importance of process evaluation, the effects which participants' beliefs have on impact evaluation, cost-effectiveness and various issues specific to self-treatment programmes for patients with asthma or other chronic diseases.

Evaluation and measurement: some dilemmas for health education

Lawrence W. Green. *American Journal of Public Health* 1977;67(2): 155–160.

This article looks at seven problems in the design and evaluation of health education projects.

1. The difficulty of designing a study which is flexible enough to be interesing but rigid enough to be scientific.

2. The dilemma between running a study which proves its theoretical point or one which gives results applicable to the real world.

3. The ways in which the beliefs of the patients (or consumers) affect the results of a programme.

4. The effects of economies of scale.

5. The importance of good timing in the parts of a programme which have an impact on its subjects.

6. The importance of good timing in evaluation.

7. The various ways of determining the budget for a programme.

This is an excellent article which clearly addresses many important issues, but gives solutions to only some of the questions it raises.

Evaluation of school health education; identifying purpose, keeping perspective

Marshall W. Kreuter and Lawrence W. Green. *Journal of School Health* 1978; April: 228–235.

A paper for those concerned with health education in schools. Compelling arguments are given for the need to evaluate school education (for professional growth and for programme survival).

The authors point out that health education programmes differ in their purposes: as with all primary prevention, success is difficult to measure objectively, which has led to behaviour change being unopposed as a standard goal, even though there is no evidence that it is always an appropriate evaluation criterion. This problem leads the authors to recommend that school health education should be evaluated at three levels: process evaluation, 'precursor evaluation' (which we have called 'impact evaluation') and outcome evaluation, with care being taken that observers are not led to expect outcome results where only impact results are available.

The social context of alcohol and drug education: implications for program evaluations

Ralph A. Weisheit. *Journal of Alcohol and Drug Education* 1983;29: 72–81.

The school alcohol and drug education field gives good examples of programmes with multiple goals. Most evaluators have focused only on the narrow goals articulated by the programme developers. Consequently, the evaluation results often suggest that the programme has failed, even though it may have been highly valued by the people running the programme and by the community within which it is run. This may lead to a loss of face for the evaluator, making it more difficult for the evaluator to recommend improvements in the programme.

Weisheit believes that alcohol education in schools is doomed to failure or very limited success. His arguments, centred around this particular problem, are relevant to any programme in which the evaluator could have an important formative role despite the programme's failure to meet its stated goals. He advocates that the evaluator use a pluralistic approach, taking into account the interests of all the groups involved (parents, school personnel, programme developers, governments, etc.). Objectives which are not stated (e.g., being seen to tackle the problem, or an improvement in student-teacher interactions) are still objectives, and are to be evaluated along with changes in knowledge and behaviour. Examples of how to do this are not given!

Readability formulas may mislead you
James W. Pichert and Peggy Elam. *Patient Education and Counselling* 1985;7:181–191.

Readability formulas alone cannot determine whether a piece of writing will be understood by its audience. For example, compare two sentences with the same meaning:

1. 'What what what he wanted cost in Middle Wallop would buy in London was amazing.'
2. 'It was amazing what could be bought in Middle Wallop for the cost in London of what he wanted'.

The first sentence scores at least as well as the second in most formal readability test, but is a lot harder to read!

Bearing in mind that formulas are not perfect, this article considers how best to improve readability. When readability formulas are used, three criteria should be observed.

1. Readability formulas should not be the sole way of assessing whether a piece of text is comprehensible.
2. The readers for whom the text is intended should be similar to those on whom the formula was statistically validated.
3. Readability formulas are valid only as a way of evaluating texts, not as a recipe for writing them.

BOOKS

Evaluation of Human Service Programs
C.C. Attkisson, W.A. Hargreaves, M.J. Horowitz and J.E. Sorensen, (eds). New York: Academic Press, 1987.

'Human service programmes' in this book designates private and public programmes designed and organized to address individual or family problems, or personal needs for growth and development, and so includes all aspects of health services including health education and health promotion.

In this book, programme evaluation is described as a form of feedback within the process of managing programmes: in other words, it is formative. The emphasis is on the need for building up skills and the capacity for evaluation at all levels from service delivery to policy making and so this book is quite large in scope and in physical size.

This volume is somewhere between a book of collected readings and a purpose written text. One or more of the editors contributes to most of the chapters, along with a number of other contributors. Some chapters are rather thickly written. Cross-references help the reader interested in one particular topic make his or her way around the volume.

Issues covered include:

- the historical context of human service delivery
- the role of evaluation in programming
- information systems and how to use them
- assessing community needs
- comparing costs and effectiveness in evaluation
- the future for program evaluation

Recommended chapters: Chapter 12—Kiresuk on Goal Attainment Scaling in its original intended form; Chapter 4—Roles and Functions of Evaluation in Human Service Programs; Chapter 5—Program Evaluation on a Shoestring Budget.

Health Education and Health Promotion Planning
Mark B. Dignan and Patricia A. Carr. Philadelphia: Lea and Febiger, 1987.

A recent publication which has already gained considerable respect from its US audience. This book represents the state of the art in health education in the US. The authors take a broad view of health education planning and seek to integrate several models of behavioural assessment such as PRECEDE, SORC and Communication Persuasion. The title is, however, somewhat misleading since there is little in the book that extends health promotion out from individual behaviour change.

The main feature of this book is that it presents the planning process as a joint endeavour between health professionals and the client community, emphasizing community analysis as a prerequisite for planning any programme. Chapter 3 provides an in-depth description of how to tackle community analysis and diagnosis (otherwise known as needs assessment). This description includes a comprehensive format for conducting a community analysis which would be particularly useful for those involved in establishing programme priorities and directing resources to areas of need.

A separate chapter on evaluation acknowledges evaluation as an activity that takes place throughout all phases of planning and implementating programmes. This includes a clear section on threats to validity and on variations on the quantitative and qualitative experimental design dichotomy.

Patient Education: An Enquiry into the State of the Art
Wendy Squyres. New York: Springer, 1980.

This book is presented as a course in the real-world application of health promotion principles for health educators. It describes the process of planning, developing and evaluating health education programmes for patients in close detail. There are numerous examples of both successful and unsuccessful programmes and exercises for the reader to work through, yet the broad political context is not lost in the detail. Green's PRECEDE model is followed and is translated into an exhaustive format for developing education programmes. The planning process is described from three perspectives: namely, the institutional, programme and client levels.

Community Health
L.W. Green and C.L. Anderson.
St Louis: Times Mirror/Mosby College Publishing, 1986.

This excellent and wide-ranging text sets out to familarize the reader with current issues in community health. The fifth edition is based on previous work of the authors and on contributions and insights from practitioners and academics from many countries. The style is clear and concise: through illuminating chapter headings and summaries the reader is guided through several perspectives including:

Part 1: the history of community health practice and theory;
Part 2: health issues for different periods in the lifespan (including maternal and child health, adolescent and adult health, aging);
Part 3: lifestyle determinants of health;
Part 4: environmental health protection;
Part 5: discusses resources and services involved in promoting community health, from the global and national levels down to personal health services.

Annotated readings and a bibliography are included in each chapter.

The PRECEDE model of health education planning is described, as is the authors' view of the relationship between health education and health promotion. Green and Anderson see health promotion as a separate domain, however, and only allow health educators to plan individual behaviour change. See our appendix for the differences between Green's model and our model of health promotion.

This book is an invaluable resource for all community health workers.

Health Education Planning: A Diagnostic Approach
L.W. Green, M.W. Kreuter, S.G. Deeds and K.B. Partridge.
Palo Alto: Mayfield Publishing, 1980.

This book has been around for a while now, yet it remains a benchmark in the growth and development of health education. This is where the PRECEDE framework for health education planning was first described.

PRECEDE is an acronym for 'predisposing, reinforcing and enabling causes in educational diagnosis and evaluation'. The philosophy underlying PRECEDE is one of voluntary behaviour change and consumer participation in planning health education interventions.

Behaviour change can occur in the target group or in a group which controls the rewards or resources which affect the health of the target group. The PRECEDE framework is based on the disciplines of epidemiology, social and behavioural sciences, administration and education. The term *education* is used eclectically as the chapter on educational strategies outlines relatively radical approaches such as community development, social planning, organizational development and social action as well as traditional education strategies such as lectures, skill development, simulations and games.

Detailed explanations of the framework and its application in community education, school health, dental health, patient education and occupational health are provided. There is also a very useful section on key terms.

This book predates the term 'health promotion'. Its major strength lies in the way the PRECEDE framework reflects a synthesis of the multiple factors which affect health and health behaviour. Its major weakness lies in its simplistic view of the structural barriers to behaviour change and its reductionist view that health problems can ultimately be reduced or minimized through simple changes in behaviour.

An excellent introductory text for those new to the field.

Patient Education and Health Promotion in Medical Care
Wendy Squyres.
Palo Alto: Mayfield Publishing, 1985.

This book follows on from an earlier introductory text (see above) which targeted those working specifically in the area of patient education. This later book is primarily for those intending to practise health promotion in medical care or clinical settings, including patient education, but covering other areas as well. The contributors are drawn from a number of professional backgrounds and each offers the benefit of their professional and personal experience.

From very early in the text, the reader is left in no doubt as to who makes the decisions and (by implication) controls the resources in clinical settings. Intending health educators in medical care organizations are urged to gain credibility early on and then use that credibility to influence the decision makers and thereby access resources, rather than promoting divisions between clinical care and health promotion.

In Chapter 1, a model for patient education and health promotion programming is proposed. This model informs the rest of the book as it puts forward the ideas that good health education services are the result of good planning and that health promotion services can be organized by levels of service: that is, the levels of the institution, of the programme and of the client.

The remainder of the book covers issues such as policy development, the health educator's roles, planning, implementing and evaluating education services. The PRECEDE model is applied to the development of protocols and teaching plans for patient and health education. Relatively new areas, such as health risk appraisal, strategies for decision making, and the role of self-care in medical care are also discussed. Numerous examples of techniques and formats are included, covering topics as diverse as: stop smoking programmes, evaluating closed-circuit hospital television, evaluating a health library and personal health assessment questionnaires.

This is a very helpful book for those who are already intending to work in medical settings. It is realistic and practical and takes the reader beyond the mechanics of health education practice to an exploration of the health educator as a change agent in an organizational setting.

Program Evaluation Kit

Morris, Lynn (ed.), Center for the Study of Evaluation, UCLA.
2nd ed. Beverly Hills: Sage Publications, 1987.

This kit consists of the following volumes:
1. Evaluator's Handbook
2. How to Focus an Evaluation
3. How to Design a Program Evaluation
4. How to Assess Program Implementation
6. How to Measure Attitudes
7. How to Measure Performance and Use Tests
8. How to Analyze Data
9. How to Communicate Evaluation Findings

Quite a well-known work, the kit is similar to our book in approach; but its focus is on the education of school children, not on health. Considerable space is given to examples of procedure and lists of further resources for educational projects. If you can wade through the examples on spelling and arithmetic, this series has a simply expressed explanation of what evaluation is, why you should do it and what you need to do in order to discharge your evaluation responsibilities. It discusses various approaches to evaluation (e.g. experimental, goal-oriented, user-oriented), and covers a range of practical questions for those who are looking at evaluation for the first time. Most helpful modules: *How to Focus an Evaluation; How to use Qualitative Methods in Evaluation; How to Calculate Statistics; How to Communicate Evaluation Findings.*

There is an earlier edition of this kit, but the second edition is better organized and reflects current evaluation concerns and practice.

Principles of Instructional Design

Robert M. Gagne and Leslie J. Briggs. 2nd ed.
New York: Holt, Rinehart and Winston, 1979.

This book describes what is essential for instructional (education) programmes to aid learning. It outlines some basic theory of the processes involved in learning and gives a detailed description of how to design, plan and carry out instructional programmes. There are sections on assessing student performance (which can be applied to various target groups) and on evaluating instructional designs. It is particularly useful to fieldworkers involved in intensive health education programmes.

Program Evaluation

Robert O. Brinkerhoff, Dale M. Brethower, Terry Hluchyj and Jeri Ridings Nowakowski. Boston: Kluwer-Nijhoff Publishing, 1983.

This is a three-part text concerned with evaluating educational programmes, although the principles can be applied to other health programmes. Evaluation is presented primarily as a tool for improving current and or future programmes, and there is an emphasis on recognizing good programme design.

A helpful reader's guide to the three sections makes it easy to look up particular issues of interest.

Part 1: Sourcebook—outlines principles of function and practice.

Part 2: Casebook—fictional examples of others' designs.

Part 3: Design Manual—gives step-by-step directions, worksheets, examples and checklists to help readers to design and carry out their own evaluations.

Quasi-Experimentation: Design and Analysis Issues for Field Settings

Thomas D. Cook and Donald T. Campbell. Boston: Houghton Mifflin, 1979.

This book should be helpful in deciding which design to use for a particular research or evaluation situation. It outlines the philosophical assumptions (often overlooked) which are involved in experimental field research and explains how these principles can be used in research settings where the strict experimental method (randomized control trial) is not feasible. Several quasi-experimental designs are presented including non-equivalent groups, interrupted time series and cohort designs, along with appropriate methods of statistical analysis for each. The requirements of the randomized control trial are also briefly outlined for those contexts in which it may be suitable. There is a good discussion of validity, particularly internal validity, which is used to compare designs.

Qualitative Evaluation Methods

M.Q. Patton. Beverley Hills: Sage Publications, 1980.

Patton emphasizes that research methods need to be selected for their ability to address the subtle nuances of given research questions and that methodological rigor is secondary to this. He explains clearly, using factual scenarios, what qualitative data are and how they can be used to provide depth and detail, either alone or in conjunction with quantitative data. This is not a how-to book, but it suggests ways of thinking about evaluation and methods, so that the evaluator has a broader choice of ways to produce valuable and valid data. There are helpful discussions of open-ended questionnaires, surveys, participants and observation.

Measurement in Health Promotion and Protection

T. Abelin, Z. J. Brzezinski and Vera D. L. Carstairs (eds).
Copenhagen: WHO Regional Publications, European Series No. 22
available from Hunter Publications, 58A Gipps St Collingwood 3066.

This comprehensive text is essential for all serious students of research and evaluation in health promotion. From the introductory chapter on concepts of health and health promotion to the exploration of methods of measurement and examples of their application, this book proves an indispensable guide, but it is in no way a book to be glanced at for a quick understanding of the subject, and there's no index to tempt the reader to do this. It reviews the major ways of measuring dimensions of health and processes of health promotion and health protection, including measures of behaviour, psychosocial status, quality of life, quality of air and water, infection, quality of care and health promotion indicators, and each example is drawn from real life.

This is the first joint publication of the International Epidemiological Association and the WHO Regional Office for Europe. It provides a guide to what has already been achieved in measurement in health promotion and a pointer as to where we need to go next. In these days of emphasis on the value of new qualitative measures, the authors hope that this book will create a greater understanding of how quantitative methods can be used for identifying problems, setting targets, and assessing progress towards these targets.

A Survey Research Handbook

Pamela L. Alrecq and R.B. Settle. Illinois: Irwin, 1985.

This is a book which clearly explains all the steps involved in survey research from design to final report. It consists of the following sections:

1. Survey planning and design.
2. Survey instrumentation (including question composition and questionnaire design).
3. Data collection and processing (including mailed questionnaires, interviews and telephone surveys).
4. Data analysis and reporting (including statistical analysis, interpretation of results and writing reports).

The emphasis in this book is definitely practical. There are summaries and checklists for on-the-job consultation (for example, a checklist for running a telephone survey). This is the sort of book you wish you'd had before you ever ran a survey and is recommended for newcomers and old hands alike.

Do It Yourself Social Research

Yoland Wadsworth. Melbourne: Victorian Council of Social Service

This book has become a bible for community groups setting out to collect data to help them assess needs and develop better services and programmes. The book is designed to take the mystique out of research and put research techniques in the hands of anyone who wants to set out to answer a question.

The style is friendly and direct, with lots of cartoons and graphics. As well as sections which cover the sort of areas you would expect to see (questionnaires, sampling, surveys, analysis and so on) there are chapters on time management and budgetting and how to communicate your research findings. A useful addition is a section called 'translations of common research language', designed to disarm those of us who usually like to hide behind a screen of jargon!

This book is highly recommended for health workers and for the community groups we work with.

Qualitative Data Analysis
Matthew B. Miles and A. Michael Huberman.
Beverly Hills: Sage Publications, 1984.

Qualitative data are attractive. Words are richer, more descriptive and (above all) more context-sensitive than numbers, and suggest interpretations of the world. However, qualitative data offer very little protection against self-delusion. Hypotheses framed in words and derived from words seem less scientific than statistical inferences, and the very fact that words are easier to manipulate than numbers makes it hard to know how much confidence to have in conclusions drawn from someone else's qualitative analysis, especially when hundreds of pages of notes have been reduced to a few brave statements.

This book takes the stance that evaluation material *can* be presented objectively without necessarily being derived or presented numerically. (The authors give their position the appealing name of 'soft-nosed logical positivism'.) The authors have done it, and in this book they have culled from their experience hundreds of designs and suggestions for clarification and objectification which could make sense of James Joyce.

Like our book, Qualitative Data Analysis is intended to help with the business of drawing conclusions, but finds itself obliged to first talk about planning. In the way in which the authors use the word, 'analysis' incorporates planning, data reduction, data display, framing of hypotheses, verification of conclusions and report writing. The authors work the word 'analysis' so hard that they may, like Humpty Dumpty in Through the Looking Glass, end up having to pay it extra; but they are right to insist that these activities cannot be separated from each other if they are to be done well.

For this reason, anyone who is hoping to gather a large amount of qualitative data (say, more than a dozen focus groups) is advised to get hold of this book before they start. It is a weighty volume (about a kilogram in hardback), but it is well organized. Its structure follows the way the authors suggest an intimidating mass of data should be treated: planning, analysis during data collection, analysis of individual cases, analysis across cases, display of the results of the analyses and drawing, verifying and documenting conclusions. It is easy to dip into the book and pull out a few paragraphs to help with a particular problem. Especially plentiful are imaginative ways of displaying data: doing this well not only helps with documentation but also suggests valuable hypotheses.

Evaluation of Health Promotion and Health Education Programs

Richard A. Windsor, Thomas Baranowski, Noreen Clark and Gary Cutter. Palo Alto, California: Mayfield Publishing, 1984.

This was one of the first books on health promotion evaluation and it is still one of the best. As well as chapters on evaluation techniques and data analysis, the authors present a chapter on how to use your evaluation to promote organisational change. After all, this is what we are all on about! The authors discuss different models of organisational change (evaluator managed models, open system models and so on) and give case examples from a range of health settings.

The chapters on process evaluation, methods of data collection and issues in data collection provide more detail than we do in our book. There is also a very useful chapter on data analysis. We recommend the section on cost-effective analysis.

The only question we can raise is whether the book is more suited to evaluation researchers in health promotion than it is to people primarily responsible for delivering programmes. The reason for this is the degree of competence in research techniques that is implied as being necessary. With sections on normal distributions, binomial distributions, chi squares and so on the novice evaluator is bound to be somewhat intimidated. Almost in anticipation of this comment, the authors include an appendix which outlines the role expectations of the entry level health educator published by the US Department of Health and Human Services.

Measurement and Evaluation in Health Education and Health Promotion

Lawrence W. Green and Frances Marcus Lewis. Palo Alto, California: Mayfield Publishing, 1986.

This book covers essentially the same material as the book by Windsor et al, which predates it, but it brings a different slant. Again, we would argue that it is not an introductory text. You have to already like evaluation or be very interested in it before you could get through much of what is contained in this book. Then you would find the authors' approach highly valuable.

There is a discussion of the different conceptual models that influence the way evaluation is conceived and conducted, for example the biomedical and public health model and the health education model. Getting the reader to question 'where they are coming from' before they start doing anything else is a good approach, particularly as evaluation is so powerful.

A feature of the book is a very good chapter on qualitative methods by Patricia Mullen and Donald Iverson. Some very difficult concepts are skillfully explained. The reader is also introduced to the complexities of this area and the different types of qualitative evaluation approaches there are to choose from in evaluation, such as goal-free evaluation and client analysis.

We particularly recommend the appendix where you will find a 'smorgasbord' of references to evaluations that have been published with different target groups, designs, settings, outcome or impact measures and health problems. This is a helpful starting point to finding out about evaluations that have been done on programmes similar to your own.

USEFUL ADDRESSES*

Australasian Epidemiological Association

The Australasian Epidemiological Association is an organisation affliated with the Public Health Association of Australia for those with a specialist interest in epidemiology. Contact via the Public Health Association (see below).

Australasian Evaluation Society

The Australasian Evaluation Society is a non-profit-making organisation for professionals involved in the practice or study of evaluation whose purpose is to improve the practice and utility of evaluation. The society's executive has no fixed abode, but the current president, Bryan Lenne, is happy to be contacted on (02) 269 5600 for advice about consultancy services or general advice relating to programme evaluation.

Australian Community Health Association

PO Box 657
Bondi Junction NSW   2022

Phone (02) 389   1433
Fax   (02) 387   5032

The Australian Community Health Association is a national organisation that supports and advocates for community health services at national, state and local levels. Its activities include ongoing information, education for members and other community health workers, research projects, and systems of standards and quality assurance for community health services. There are branches in six states, and a national office in Sydney.

Australian Institute of Health

GPO Box 570
Canberra ACT 2601

*Information supplied here was correct in May 1990.

242

Phone   (062)   43   5000
Fax   (062)   57   1470

The Australian Institute of Health is a statutory authority. It has a national role in coordinating and collecting health-related statistics and conducting and promoting research into health status and health services in Australia. The AIH is also involved in evaluating several major health initiatives including the National Better Health Programme.

HEAPS (Health Education and Promotion System)

National Coordinator
Victoria College, Rusden Campus
662 Blackburn Road, Clayton, Victoria 3168

Phone   (03)   542   7338
Fax   (03)   544   7413

HEAPS is a national database of health promotion programmes and resources developed by health workers in Australia. It is jointly funded by the Commonwealth and state departments of health. HEAPS is part of the Medline database and can be searched for programmes and resources relating to your area of interest.

To search the HEAPS database you will need to carry out a Medline search, available from most hospital and university or college libraries. Ask the librarian to help you. If you do not have access to a major library contact your area health promotion coordinator or your state or territory HEAPS coordinator, through your state department of health. Failing that, contact the national co-ordinator. There are phone numbers below, but these are not staffed at all times.

To register a programme with HEAPS, again, contact your area health promotion coordinator for a form which asks you to describe the programme and then return the form through your area coordinator to your state HEAPS coordinator.

State/Territory HEAPS coordinator Phone Numbers

ACT	(062)	45	4244
NSW	(02)	217	5933
NT	(089)	20	3370
QLD	(07)	234	0906
SA	(08)	226	6053
TAS	(002)	30	3776
VIC	(03)	616	7449
WA	(09)	222	2040

Public Health Association of Australia

GPO Box 2204
Canberra ACT 2601

Phone   (062)   85   2373
Fax   (062)   82   5438

PHA is a non-political organisation which acts as an advocate for public health concerns, encourages research and information exchange in areas related to public health and promotes the education and development of public health workers. Membership of PHA is open to anyone with an interest in public health.

There are PHA branch offices in each state. Contact the Canberra office for more information. The Canberra office can also provide local contact numbers for the Australasian Epidemiological Association (AEA), a smaller group which is affiliated with PHA.

Appendix 1
ALTERNATIVE APPROACHES TO HEALTH PROMOTION PLANNING

Some readers will have recognized that in discussing the causal pathways of health problems and how they might be counteracted we have slightly modified the definitions of predisposers, enablers and reinforcers as originally put forward by Lawrence Green and his colleagues (PRE-CEDE).[1] This appendix compares our approach to the original model. We have kept this explanation separate so that it does not distract from the main message of Chapters 2 and 3.

The reason why Green's terms have been modified in this book is that in his original model the focus was on changing a risk factor that was usually stated in behavioural terms. To some extent this also determined the kind of factors likely to be considered as part of the causal pathway— the predisposers, enablers and reinforcers.

We have retained and adapted these terms because we want health promotion and health education professionals to be able to apply Green's important advance in health promotion planning to the analysis of so-called non-behavioural factors that influence a health problem as well as behavioural factors.

This corresponds to an expansion of thought about what health promotion should attempt to achieve. These non-behavioural factors might be health laws, incentives, environmental regulations and so on. The framework put forward by Green et al has been successfully used to tackle the analysis of these areas and to provide a systematic planning approach.

In order to show how this approach builds on the PRECEDE model, a brief description of the original model is given.

Background to Green's Model

Health education has been described by Green et al as the voluntary adoption of behaviour conducive to health.[1,2] PRECEDE (or predisposing, reinforcing and enabling causes in educational diagnosis and evaluation) was devised as a way of assessing health education needs in a community setting. The five basic steps in PRECEDE include the social diagnosis; the epidemiological diagnosis; the behavioural diagnosis; and the administrative diagnosis. These five steps combine to bring rigor, rationality and organisation to programme design. PRECEDE draws on many disciplines to analyse the social concerns, the health problems and the behavioural and non-behavioural factors contributing to those health problems in a community. Unhealthy behaviours are further analysed for their predisposing, enabling and reinforcing factors. It is these factors which become the focus of a health education intervention which is always aimed at the voluntary adoption of healthy behaviour. When a change in behaviour needs to be preceded or supported by organizational, environmental, legislative or economic change (the non-behavioural factors), then the process becomes one of health promotion strongly supported by health education. In either case, whether health education or health promotion, the voluntary adoption of healthy behaviour is paramount.

Health Promotion Model

In this book we have employed the PRECEDE framework but expanded it to assess the *health promotion* needs of a community, analysing non-behavioural as well as behavioural risk factors. This means that the predisposing, enabling and reinforcing factors outlined in the educational diagnosis are now applied to both types of risk factors. To do this the definitions of predisposing, enabling and reinforcing factors have had to be broadened to give greater weight and emphasis to the structural factors contributing to the health problem. This means that depending on the causal pathway, action can be taken on behavioural or non-behavioural factors contributing to the health problem; and the further analysis of those risk factors does not assume a behavioural component.

For example, in analysing the health problem of child pedestrian accidents we come up against environmental and legislative factors which, along with the familiar knowledge, attitude and behaviour, contribute to the health problem. The way in which they contribute can be usefully analysed using the PRECEDE framework. A lack of pedestrian crossings, or a lack of legal obligation for drivers to stop for children crossing the road, can be described as a factor which *enables* conditions that lead to accidents—these are just as important *enabling factor*s as a lack of road-crossing skills in children. It is not necessary to posit a direct link between installing crossings and voluntary behaviour change amongst drivers to be able to use the PRECEDE framework to analyse the problem and suggest solutions. Although Green's model was largely motivated by behavioural science, its extension to cover non-behavioural influences in health does not compromise its theoretical legitimacy.

Practical Differences between PRECEDE and Needs Assessment

While there are direct parallels between the steps in PRECEDE and the steps in **needs assessment,** the essential difference lies in our retention of the non-behavioural as well as the behavioural risk factors—see Figure 29.

Table 14. *The different definitions of predisposing, enabling and reinforcing factors.*

Factor	Green et al[1]	Our Model
Predisposing	Any characteristic of a patient, consumer, student, or community that motivates behaviour related to health	Any characteristic of an individual, a community or an environment that predisposes behaviour or other conditions related to health. Includes knowledge, belief and attitude, but may include other factors such as socioeconomic status. These factors can predispose conditions which lead to ill health or conditions which lead to good health, e.g. lack of knowledge of the sexual transmission of HIV predisposes people to practising unsafe sex
Enabling	Any characteristic of the environment that facilitates health behaviour, and any skill or resource required to attain the behaviour	Any characteristic of an individual, group or environment that facilitates health behaviour or other conditions affecting health, including any skill or resource required to attain that condition. Enabling factors can facilitate conditions that lead to ill health (e.g. lack of easy access to condoms) or conditions that lead to good health (e.g. availability of healthy take-away food)
Reinforcing	Rewards or punishments following or anticipated as a consequence of a health behaviour	Any reward or punishment or any feedback following or anticipated as a consequence of a health behaviour

Figure 28.   *Summarizing the conceptual differences in approach*

Green, Kreuter, Partridge and Deeds.[1]

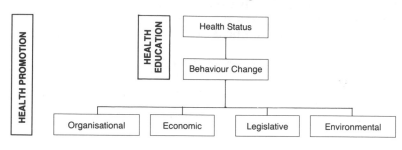

Our Model

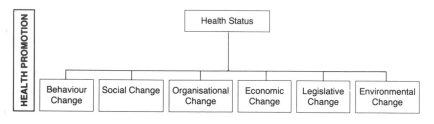

Figure 29.   *Stepwise comparison of PRECEDE*
and Needs Assessment

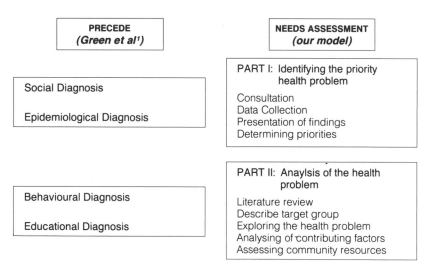

Figure 30.   *Stepwise Comparison of*
                        Programme Planning approaches

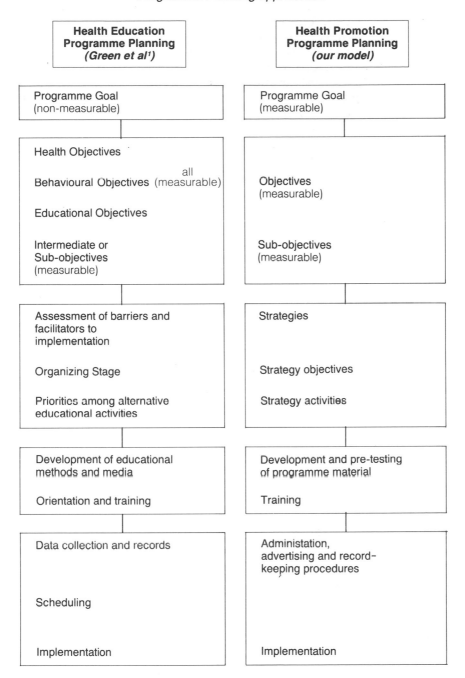

Practical Differences in Programme Planning

In programme planning there are two main differences between the models. For a start, our approach uses a measurable goal as well as measurable objectives. We believe it is important to be able to measure the goal of a programme to see whether it is having an effect on the health problem of interest. Also, in our model a goal can be set at any point on the causal pathway. It need not automatically follow that the goal addresses the health problem, the objectives address the risk factors, and the sub-objectives address the contributing factors. A linear summary of the two models is set out in Figure 30.

References

1. Green LW, Kreuter M W, Deeds S G, Partridge K B. *Health Education Planning A Diagnostic Approach*. Palo Alto: Mayfield Publishing, 1980.
2. Green L W, Anderson C L. *Community Health*. St Louis: Times Mirror/ Mosby College Publishing, 1986.

Index

251

readability of material 70–2, 73
reinforcing factors *glos*, 33–4
reports 26–7, 154–5
response rates 147–8
risk factor *glos*, 33–5
  and planning 44–6
risk markers *glos*, 33–4

S

sample *glos*
  size 26, 135–7
  types 133–5
SMOG formula (readability) 70–1, 73
snowball sample 135
social scientists 197–8
Southern Vales Community Services
Research Unit 26–7
staff
  and evaluation 11–12
  training 52–4
standard deviation 152
statistical significance 124–5
statisticians 196
strategy activities 51, 52, 53, 57
strategy objectives 42–3, 51, 52, 53, 57
  and evaluation 44

study design 223–5
sub-objectives *glos*, 42, 43
  and contributing risk factor
    44–6
  and evaluation 44
  need to specify 46–9
support networks
  measuring 112–13
surveys *glos*, 132–3
  annotated bibliography 239–40
  choosing a sample 134–7
  planning 137–40
systematic sample 134–5

T

target groups *glos*
  describing 30–1
  and evaluation 10
time series evaluation *glos*
  in non-equivalent groups 122
  in single group 121

U

users, of evaluation 90–1